BLACK SUICIDE

Published in the United States by
Beckham Publications Group, Inc.
P.O. Box 4066, Silver Spring, MD 20914

ISBN: 978-0-9823876-0-3

Library of Congress Control Number: 2009922866

BLACK SUICIDE

THE TRAGIC REALITY of America's Deadliest Secret

Alton R. Kirk, PhD

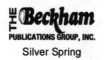

PUBLICATIONS GROUP, INC.

Silver Spring

to
Blake Alton Riley
My Grandson

Contents

Foreword

Donna Holland Barnes, PhD

Dr. Alton Kirk's *Black Suicide: The Tragic Reality of America's Deadliest Secret* should be read by anyone even distantly interested in suicide among the black population. This book is long past due only because it is a capsule of education on suicide—like a pill—you read and feel much better about understanding suicide in the African-American communities. Few people understand this topic better than Dr. Kirk. He is well aware of the history, the present issues, and what lies ahead for us in this field of suicidology.

Dr. Kirk has been highly published on the topic since the seventies—before the rates of suicide among African-American males became a public issue and declared a public health problem. In 1975, he presented a paper at the American Association of Suicidology "Black Suicide: Area of Neglect by Social Scientist." In the presentation, he outlined the lack of research in this arena, the lack of concern and the lack of emphasis by major researchers in the field of suicidology. In fact, the majority of his presentations at major conferences were on the issue of black suicide right up to the present day. He never lost interest in the subject and kept up with everything written on the topic.

In 1977, Dr. Kirk was one of the first to frame the argument that stress in black males is a correlation to suicidal behavior, attempts and completions. He argued that many social, physical, political, economical and psychological forces in the system contribute to stress among black males. These systemic forces are much more prevalent in black communities.

Dr. Kirk joined organizations that were springing up in the mid nineties and attended the meetings—specifically Suicide Prevention Action Group (formerly known as Suicide Prevention Advocacy Group) founded by Jerry and Elsie Weyrauch in Atlanta, Georgia after the lost of their daughter to suicide. SPAN was one of the first, if not the first, organizations founded by survivors of suicide where suicide prevention was its primary focus and who made quite an impact on the suicide prevention movement as we know it today. During a SPAN meeting led by the Weyrauchs and attended mostly by white families who have lost someone to suicide, Dr. Kirk stood up and asked, "Where are the black families?" and "Have you reached out to them?" At that time in 1997, Dr. Kirk knew the rates of suicide among African Americans had increased substantially as mentioned in Chapter 2. And if the rates increased, why then, was everyone in the room white? What is wrong with this picture? he said to himself.

About a year later, he attended another national meeting with SPAN. Doris Smith from Atlanta and I—who both lost sons to suicide—were the only two blacks in the room (we thought). We were sitting up front as the meeting came to a close. I turned around and noticed a black man in the back standing up against the wall. I turned and said, "Doris, there is another black in the room... there's a black man back there!!!" After the meeting, Doris and I could not wait to meet him and introduce ourselves so that we could have a good discussion about suicide among African Americans and the lack of support from other blacks to get involved with suicide prevention and intervention.

Around the same time, the organization of NOPCAS was beginning to form. Dr. Kirk was the very first one we asked to join our board. He has been with us since 1999 and certainly a strong force for NOPCAS. Our board is now made up of 18 members nationally with a scientific advisory board that is also national. I didn't know how we could organize a national organization whose primary focus is suicide prevention and intervention among people of color and *not* have Dr.Kirk onboard.

Because of his strong force and determination to bring attention to suicide among blacks, he was actually a lone star when it came to evaluating what was written about suicide among African Americans. In the beginning years of the 70s—not much was written. Kirk had something to say about all that which was written. He would read it, review it, publish his review, and keep moving. Some of his reviews were highly critical because the research that was claimed to be conducted was done loosely or not scientific enough. He got into heated discussions with white researchers who claimed to know what they were talking about while attending national meetings. Dr. Kirk was being a rebel and took this position: if you are going to tell the story, tell it right!

Black Suicide: The Tragic Reality of America's Deadliest Secret by Dr. Alton Kirk tells the story with more reliability. This book is not based on assumptions. It is based on history, his own research and true testaments from those who have lost someone to suicide. It's the stories at the end of the book that drive it to the home plate. It brings all the statistics and the theories to life.

Donna Holland Barnes, PhD
President and Executive Director
National Organization for People of Color Against Suicide
Washington, DC
http://www.nopcas.com

Acknowledgments

I offer my heartfelt appreciation for the many individuals and groups who have contributed directly and indirectly to the completion of this book. First, I have to thank my family, Gerri, Kristi, Julian and Blake whose love and support allowed me to move forward on this book.

Vicki L. Oberlin and Charles F. Upshaw whose help I have had since the inception of this book— thank you for your inspiration. You were there when I needed it most. Mary "Pete" Martin helped to keep the dream alive, pushed me to meet deadlines, and did the initial typing of the manuscript—many thanks. To Mary Langston for her typing and conceptual assistance, especially in the development of the "Wheel of Destructive Behaviors," thank you for your long hours of endeavor. Thank you also to Gail Garber (Mrs. "G") for her initial editing and typing of the manuscript. I could always depend on her helpful suggestions and recommendations. Thanks to Dr. Alex E. Crosby of the Centers for Disease Control and Prevention (CDC), for his consultations throughout the years. A very special thanks to my dear friends of many years, Dr. Ruth E. Dennis and L. John Key with whom I have presented papers and attended conferences regarding black suicide and other forms of destructive behaviors.

Thanks to my family of organizations that deal with the research, understanding, causes, prevention and postvention of suicide: The National Organization for People of Color Against Suicide (NOPCAS) and its President and Executive Director, Dr. Donna Barnes, and the Michigan Association for Suicide Prevention and its president, my good friend and colleague, Larry Lewis. I am grateful to NOPCAS for giving me the honor and privilege of serving on its board of directors. We have all certainly functioned as a family in our work toward preventing suicide and providing services to survivors via Survivors of Suicide groups (SOS). I thank all of you for your support throughout the years.

Thank you also to the American Association of Suicidology (AAS) where I got my start more than 35 years ago. This organization provided invaluable training and exposure to the most notable scholars in the field of suicidology including its founding president, Dr. Edwin Shneidman. AAS honored me in 1977, by awarding the "Young Contributors Award," later renamed the "Edwin Shneidman Award" for my innovative research in black suicide. Dr. Lanny Berman, executive director, has been instrumental in the growth of AAS since the national office was moved from Denver, Colorado to Washington, D.C.

I thank my most influential professors at Michigan State University where I received my doctorate in clinical psychology: my advisors, Dr. Robert A. Zucker, along with Dr. Bertram P. Karon, and Dr. Dozier W. Thornton, whose contributions to my growth as a psychologist are immeasurable.

A very special thank-you goes to North Carolina Central University and its psychology department: Drs. Howard Wright, Carol C. Bowie, and Marion D. Thorpe. They allowed me to dream that I could become a clinical psychologist during a time (1950s) of die-hard racial segregation and discrimination.

I apologize to those of you whose names I may have omitted because of limited space. Your support, love and encouragement are deeply appreciated.

Finally, thanks to Barry Beckham and his staff at the Beckham Publications Group for making the dream of this book a reality.

Introduction

Edward Arlington Robinson's poem, "Richard Cory," sowed the seed for this book when I was a sophomore in high school. I read the poem in a literature class and it ended in suicide when Cory "went home and put a bullet through his head." My friends, Frank, Bob and I laughed when we first heard this poem.

We knew at least two things for sure. One, Richard Cory was a white man; black people did not commit suicide. Two, Cory had to have been crazy since he had everything going for him. He was rich, well dressed, admired by people, and even envied by some others who wanted to be in his place. In spite of having all these things going for him, Cory took his own life.

I felt then, as did most people in the black community, that suicide was a "white thing"; black people didn't commit suicide. We were too strong and too tough to do such a thing. Wicked people had brought our ancestors to this country by force and enslaved them for centuries. Black people survived that period of dehumanization with a sense of powerlessness and rage. Even after the end of slavery, the larger society in which we lived forced black people into a segregated world in which we faced racial discrimination on a daily basis. In spite of these painful, adverse conditions, black people survived, in part, because of their toughness, their strong religious faith, and their strong family ties, which we believed kept us from doing such a "weak-minded white thing" as committing suicide. That is what I thought as a high school sophomore and well after that.

I was not alone. As I grew older, I put away such childish thoughts.

In 1999, Dr. David Satcher, then the U.S. surgeon general, issued a momentous report, "Call to Action to Prevent Suicide." It recognized suicide as a public health problem by a national public official for the first time and brought suicide to the public's attention, as it had not been done before. The report states:

> Suicide is a serious public health problem. In 1997, the year for which the most recent statistics were available, suicide was the eighth leading cause of mortality in the United States, responsible for nearly 31,000 deaths. This number is more than 50 percent higher than the number of homicides in the U.S. in the same year (around 20,000 in 1996). Yet, people learn of the latest homicides through the media on a daily basis, while media reports on suicides occur much less. Many people fail to realize that far more Americans die from suicide than from homicide. Each year in the U.S., approximately 500,000 people require emergency-room treatment because of attempted suicide. Suicidal behavior typically occurs in the presence of mental

or substance abuse disorders—illnesses that impose their own direct suffering. Suicide is an enormous trauma for millions of Americans who experience the loss of someone close to them. The nation must address suicide as a significant public health problem and put into place national strategies to prevent loss of life and the suffering suicide causes.

Only in recent years have black people begun to recognize that suicide is a major problem for them. Suicide within the black community exists in far greater numbers and for a longer period than many people realize.

If you just look at the suicide rate in general, you might be misled. For example, the suicide rate is highest among white males, while the overall suicide rate for blacks in general is relatively low. However, when you look at age- specific suicides, the suicide rate for young black men is much higher than you might expect. This anomaly has existed for many years. In the late 1960s and 1970s, there was a great deal of suicide research addressing the high suicide rate among young black males. In the late 1980s and early 1990s, there was a significant decline in the interest and research of black suicide. Only a few people kept the issue of black suicide as a viable social issue.

In the late 1990s there was a resurgence of interest and research in black suicide. A larger than ever number of black social scientists and researchers was interested in black suicide: Crystal Barksdale, Donna Barnes, Alex E. Crosby, Kevin E. Early, Sean Joe, Samantha Matlin, Sherry Molock, and Rupa Purl. This younger generation of researchers has added a great deal to the body of knowledge regarding the understanding and prevention of black suicide. Even with this sudden rush of new research, one thing remained constant: black suicides among males occur at an earlier age than for whites and other ethnic groups.

There was a change in 1999 in the way researchers and doctors recorded their studies, which makes the comparison of data prior to 1999 somewhat problematic. The fact remains as reported by Crosby and Molock in 2006, "African-American adolescents and young adults have the highest number and the highest rate of suicide of any age group of African Americans. Suicide was the third leading cause of death among African-American people aged 15 to 19 years, fourth among those aged 20 to 29 years, and eighth among those aged 30 to 39. Among African-American adolescents and young adults, males have the highest rates of suicide. During early 1990s, the suicide rates among African-American males aged 15 to 24 were rising. The rates peaked in 1993 at 20.2 per one hundred thousand, then began a steady decline to a rate 11.6 per hundred thousand (42.6 percent decrease) in 2002."

While the low overall black suicide rate may seem to represent small numbers, any one suicide is unacceptable. Black people are killing themselves at a rate higher than ever. We must do all that we can to stop this from happening.

In this book, I will briefly discuss several theories on suicide. I will also examine social, economic, religious, political, psychological, and racial forces as factors contributing to black suicide.

For more than 35 years I have been studying, teaching, and researching the literature in the area of black suicide. However, I have been profoundly affected by working directly with suicidal black people in my clinical practice. I was able to help most of them; others I was not, some of them committed suicide. The pains of these experiences are very difficult to describe.

Spending time with the family members of those who died by suicide, rehashing what we did, what we didn't do, seconding guessing ourselves, looking for answers, dealing with guilt, embarrassment, anger and shame are all part of the process during the aftermath of a suicide. Attending funerals, talking with ministers, deciding what to say and how to say it to family members, and friends are all issues that I have tried to address. Never being adequately prepared to respond to the question, "Why didn't you save her (or him)? You are supposed to be the suicide expert." These are all painful experiences that I have endured while working in this field.

I hope this book will add to the growing body of information about black suicide and contributes in some way to help us significantly reduce the number of black suicides. In a section on survivors, those who are left behind after a suicide, you will read what these survivors have to say in their own words about how the suicides of their loved ones have affected their lives. They tell us how their loved one's suicide disrupted their lives, destroyed their dreams, and left them in a state of turmoil and pain as they live their lives as survivors of suicide.

I recommend and suggest ways to help reduce the number of suicides, as well as other behaviors

that are destructive to black people. The following
declaration appears on a plaque in the Charles H.
Wright Museum of African-American History in
Detroit Michigan:

> "Over time, people of African descent
> have changed how they wished to be called.
> In the 1700s and earlier, sons and
> daughters of (Africans) were common. By
> the 1830s, Colored Americans, People of
> Color and Afro Americans were used. By
> the early 1900s, a younger generation felt
> that Negro was a new term of pride. In
> the 1960s, a new younger generation felt
> that Black or Black American was the
> better term. Today, many people use the
> term African American, coming almost
> full circle to the 1700s."

I have chosen to use the term "black" in this
book. I am aware that many people use the term
African American. To me, the terms are
interchangeable.

Alton R. Kirk

Section I

Theories of Suicide

• Sociological Theories   • Psychological Theories

The basic theories of suicide come from sociology, psychology and psychiatry. One of the earliest and best-known suicide theories derives from the French sociologist Emil Durkheim. In 1897, Durkheim was the first to study suicide systematically, one of the first persons to do so. His contributions to the field have had a major influence on subsequent sociological and psychological theories of suicide. Sigmund Freud was another pioneering suicide theorist. Freud provided the framework for psychoanalytic and psychological suicide theories.

There are no established historical theories of black suicide. The relatively few studies of black suicide used the basic theories developed by Durkheim and Freud to examine black suicide.

Sociological Theories of Suicide

Durkheim fully described three types of suicide. One is egoistic, where the individual is insufficiently integrated into one's society. Another is altruistic, where one is so integrated into one's society that one sacrifices one's self, as in the case of a soldier on the battlefield. Durkheim's third description of suicide is anomic, in which a great economic depression, or increase in sudden wealth causes an adjustment in a person's life. The fourth, and least known of Durkheim's theories, is that of fatalistic suicide "derived from excessive regulations." Durkheim found this type in "persons with futures pitilessly blocked and passions violently choked by oppressive discipline." Durkheim made only passing references to fatalistic suicide because he felt it had "so little contemporary importance" and provided too few examples. However, he acknowledged its possible historical antecedents in terms of slave suicides and "all suicides attributable to excessive physical or moral despotism."

Durkheim's work on suicide influenced Henry and Short and they developed postulates of their own. Most notably, they observed that the suicide rate of a population varies inversely with the strength of the relational systems of the members. The strength of the relational system of the members of a population varies directly with the external restraints placed on their behavior. It follows that the external restraints placed on the behavior of individuals vary inversely with the societal members' status.

Given the low social and economic status of black people in the segregated United States at the time of Henry and Short's research, one would believe that white suicide rates would exceed that of blacks. One might also conclude that the suicide rate of males would exceed that of females; and high-income groups would have suicide rates higher than low-income groups. As Henry and Short would later point out, suicides do not follow such uniform trends. This is especially true for suicides among black people. When looking at suicide statistics it is important to look at age-specific groups to get a realistic picture. There have been some studies, which report the suicide rates for black males between the ages of 18-24 have at times exceeded that of whites in that age group (Hendin 1969, Kirk 1976). There are many other sociological studies regarding black suicide.

Psychological Theories of Suicide

Most psychological theories of suicide stem from Sigmund Freud's theory of depression and retroflexed rage. This notion states that no one kills oneself who does not wish to kill someone else. Alfred Adler built upon Freud's theory. He believed that suicide was a retaliatory act.

Bertram Karon, a professor of psychology at Michigan State University, along those same lines says in his article in the *Journal of Individual Psychology*, "Suicide may best be understood as an aggressive retaliatory act toward significant figures in the patient's present life, or toward fantasies of significant figures in the patient's past. The primary motivating fantasy includes the wish to hurt someone else and the belief that suicide would accomplish this end. The patient has an image of how sorry or guilty people will be if he dies."

The historical theories briefly described above provide the foundation for almost all contemporary theories and research and consequent treatment of suicidal patients. Either most contemporary theorists and practitioners embrace one or more of these theories in total or at the very least, derive their own theories directly and entirely from these earlier conclusions.

While these general theories provide a basis for our understanding of suicide, there are those, including me, who believe that the variances among cultures are significant enough to warrant modification of the older suicide theories on a culture-by-culture basis. Based upon my own research, as well as on experience in my clinical practice, I have found that as foundations some of these theories can be very helpful. However, I take issue with the implication that health professional can apply any, or all, to all cultures, or ethnic groups.

It is significant that you keep in mind that Eurocentric practitioners originated these historical theories. The error made by most researchers on black suicide has been to apply Eurocentric theories to the black population without considering the difference between European and American societies. For example, while Durkheim asserted a fourth theory, "fatalistic suicide," he deemed it generally insignificant. From the Eurocentric perspective, this was an accurate assumption. Applied to American society with its history of slavery and continuing issue of racism, this omission distorts both causal and results-oriented conclusions in the study of black suicide.

There are, in fact, American researchers who have recognized this significance and have attempted to tweak Durkheim's theories to make them pertinent and applicable to the American experience. These researchers from the fields of psychology, sociology and psychiatry are all white males who have done research on black suicide in American.

While there have been few early works on black suicide by black psychiatrists like Charles R. Prudhomme, whose 1938 article, "The Problem of Suicide in the American Negro" appeared in the *Psychoanalytic Review*, it was not until the late 1960s and the 1970s that black researchers began to make a significant impact on the study of black suicide. Those earlier researchers include L. Banks, J. Bush, Robert Davis, Ruth E. Dennis, Alton R. Kirk, Sherrie Molock, Alvin Poussaint, and Bobby Wright.

These researchers were more culturally sensitive to the psychological, social, cultural and racial variables that significantly contributed to black suicidal behaviors. Their research added tremendously to the body of knowledge of black suicide, which helped to improve the treatment techniques and protocol for black people with suicidal problems. Their research has also added to improvements in suicide prevention methods for black people.

Fortunately, there is a younger group of black scholars and researchers. These include Alex Crosby, Sean Joe and Sherrie Molock, among others, who are expanding on previous research and adding significantly to the body of knowledge about suicidal behaviors of black people and suicide prevention among black people.

Black Suicide in America

•Historical Overview •Violence Within The Black
Community • Victim Precipitated Homicide
•Mental Illness and Suicide
•Religion and Suicide

Suicide among black people has always been a
part of the black experience, especially the black
experience in America. Black people have always
occupied a unique position in the society since they
are the only race introduced to this country as
slaves. When Europeans kidnapped Africans and
brought them here on slave ships, many Africans
decided that they did not want to be slaves and
starved themselves to death on the ships. Others
jumped overboard, choosing death by drowning, or
by sharks trailing the slave ships. Black Americans
have been, and continue to be, in a state of denial
about suicide.

Until recently, social scientists have focused on
the high homicide rate among black people—the
high rate of assaults, domestic violence and black-
on-black crime, in general. In fact, *Ebony* magazine
(August 1979) published a special issue on black-

on-black crime: the causes, the consequences, the cures.

Violence within the Black Community

Throughout the years I have heard it said that "blacks are their own worst enemy." Have you ever heard such an assertion? If you are black, and of a certain age, you may remember this rhyme: "If you're light, you're all right, if you're brown stick around, but if you're black, stay the hell back." There were other derogetory rhymes. Here is one that refers to women's light versus dark skin color and their acceptability, "My gal is red hot, your gal ain't dooly squat." And, of course, there was always "playing the dozens."

During the 1940s, 1950s, 1960s and later, terms used by black people toward other black people like "little black sambo," "you black dog," "sorry black-ass nigger" were terms that would surely provoke a confrontation that would often result in arguments, fights, and far too frequently, homicides.

In the book, *The Human Side of Homicide*, I make this reference regarding an article that appeared in *Ebony* magazine in 1979, which stated that more blacks were killed by other blacks in 1977 than were killed in the entire nine-year Vietnam War. During that year, 5,734 black people were victims of other black people. The Vietnam War claimed 5,711 black lives. Black self-destruction and especially black homicide had become an increasing problem among the nation's black population. However, there was a decline in the national black homicide rate following the

1980s. In fact, the suicide rate is now higher than the homicide rate among black Americans.

What is the cause of this intra-racial discrimination and hostility that often leads to black-on-black violence? One possible explanation is that of repressed anger and hostility toward white people who are historically viewed as the oppressors. This repressed anger and hostility is too often misdirected toward those with whom black people live and socialize. For example, a black man may be angry and upset with a white boss at work. He fears that he has too much to lose—job, family, jail—if he expresses his anger toward the boss. Therefore, when he comes home, he expresses his anger and his hostility toward his spouse, his partner, or his children.The theory of repressed anger and hosititily toward white people as the opressor is one of many theories that have been offered to explain back intra-racial violence.

Victim Precipitated Homicide

What professionals regarded as "victim precipitated homicide" is, in fact, a form of suicide. Victim precipitated homicide occurs when one person provokes another to kill him or her. Richard Seiden addressed this form of suicide in 1972 and offered the following example of such behavior. A black man goes into a bar frequented by white off-duty police officers, makes threats, reaches in his coat as if to retrieve a weapon that he does not have, and a white police officer shoots him to death. Some of these deaths were officially recorded as justifiable homicides.

Pundits in recent years have called such deaths "suicide by cops." Did the police officer die? Was the cop's life ended? No, but the victim's life was lost. This is an indirect way of bringing about one's own demise, a form of suicide—victim precipitated suicide.

Mental Illness and Suicide

Black people, like other groups in our society, suffer from a wide range of mental illnesses, especially depression. Depression is the most common psychological state associated with suicide. One significant difference in the treatment of mental illness between white and black people lies in the lack of treatment, or poor quality of treatment that black people receive.

The National Mental Health Association in 2000 stated in a publication, "2.5 million Americans have bipolar disorder also called manic-depressive illness. A person with bipolar disorder can go from feeling very high (called mania) to feeling very low (depression). With proper treatment, people can control these mood swings and lead fulfilling lives. While the rate of bipolar disorder may be the same among African American as it is among other Americans, African Americans are less likely to receive a diagnosis and therefore, treatment for this illness." The article states further, "Most African Americans with bipolar disorder are going undiagnosed and untreated." The publication lists several factors that have contributed to African Americans not receiving help for bipolar disorder and other mental illnesses.

They include:

- A mistrust of health professionals, based in part on historically higher-than-average institutionalization of African Americans with mental illness; and on previous mistreatments, like such tragic events as the Tuskegee syphilis study.

- Cultural barriers between many doctors and their patients. Reliance on family and religious community, rather then mental health professionals, during times of emotional distress.

- A tendency to talk about physical problems, rather than discuss mental symptoms, or to mask symptoms with substance abuse or other medical conditions.

- Socioeconomic factors which can limit access to medical and mental health care. About 25 percent of African Americans do not have health insurance.

- Continued misunderstanding and stigma about mental illness.

Again, it is important to remember that until recent years, there were very few black psychiatrists, clinical psychologists, and other mental health professionals trained to provide psychotherapy to black people. As a result, the black population is greatly underserved in the area of mental illness. When white and other non-black psychotherapists treated them, the quality of treatment was questionable due to the limited understanding of black culture and how black people were racially perceived.

Clearly shown in the book, *In the Beginning Even the Rat Was White,* by Robert Guthrie, is the influence of racism on psychology. In his book, Guthrie illustrates how the field of psychology established and maintained a healthy alliance with several racist themes. Guthrie also presents an historical analysis of the background of mental testing, with emphasis on the concept of the "Mulatto hypotheses" of the 1920s. Here he provides evidence that clearly illustrates the obsession of early white American psychologists with the testing of black people. He substantiates his position that the so- called scientific intelligence tests "were used to replace anthropometric attempts to establish racial stratifications which placed blacks and other ethnic minorities in the lowest possible positions."

Another black scholar, clinical psychologist Bobby Wright, showed how the influence of racism might affect psychology and consequently the treatment of black people in psychotherapy. He maintains: "One of the most difficult tasks of a Black scholar is to be able to analyze the influence of racism on Black behavior and attitudes, and at the same time escape the almost irresistible Western scholarship protective barrier, namely 'the analysis of the victim.' There is no question that this 'analysis of the victim'methodology has been a major 'scientific'development of White scientists because it effectively leads away from the cause of Black's condition which is White pathology."

Religion and Suicide

Religion has always been a major force in the history of black people. Religion was perhaps the source of strength that black people needed to maintain their lives in constant repressive circumstances. Religion was a source of hope, something to look forward to, to make present life tolerable. It provided the expectation of a heavenly home after death. For these reasons, religion has for many, many years served as a deterrent to suicide for many black people. The common belief is that committing suicide will prevent one from going to heaven. While I have not found any theological data to support this belief, I respect those who believe it and view it as a positive cultural reason to keep black people from committing suicide.

While we generally accept death as a part of the life cycle, no other form of death affects us as strongly as death by suicide. It hurts when we lose a loved one or friend who dies from an illness. Accidental deaths are also painful, as are deaths by homicides. In each of these forms of death, we generally see them as causes beyond the control of the deceased individual.

Death by suicide is far more difficult to accept. We find it hard to believe that anything could be so bad, or so painful that one would make the decision to take one's own life. We say things like, "My God, it couldn't have been that bad," or "Why didn't Clarence come to me," or "Sarah was such a smart and attractive young woman, she could have easily found another man."

Black people have grown up, for the most part, believing that persons who committed suicide would not go to heaven. In spite of these beliefs and taboo, there are far more black suicides than many of us are aware of. Black suicides leave thousands of survivors in a painfully confused emotional state that is difficult to understand, accept, or express.

Grief of a suicide death is unlike any other type of grief. Guilt, anger, hurt, confusion, embarrassment and social stigma are a few of the many gut-wrenching issues that suicide survivors face. The issue of "why" can never be satisfactorily answered for suicide survivors. If suicide survivors do not adequately address, or deal with these issues in a timely manner, or do not receive support, they may become at high risk for physical ailments, emotional distress, serious psychological problems, like clinical depression, and even the risk of suicide itself.

All emotions become more intensified for the survivor after a death by suicide. Survivors may experience feelings of guilt, fear, anger, disgust, denial, abandonment, rage, confusion, or even a desire for death itself to join the deceased loved one, or to rid oneself of seemingly intolerable physical, emotional and psychological pains.

The Impact of Suicide

We are all affected to some extent by suicide—emotionally, religiously, socially, and economically. If you have not lost anyone close to you by suicide then you may never fully understand the hurt, the anguish, the heartache, the despair that survivors of suicide experience. However, you will gain a better understanding of the survivors' continual painful experiences when you read in Section II what survivors have to say about their experiences after the suicide of their loved ones.

In the early years, black people were in denial about back suicide. Many black people viewed suicide as a "white thing." My colleagues often criticized me for wasting time studying such a phenomenon as "black suicide." They suggested to me on many occasions that if I wanted to do something meaningful, I should focus on black homicide, which in those years was prevalent and received more publicity and scholarly attention than black suicide.

I took the position then, and maintain it now, that there is a destructive behavior cycle among black people—especially black males. There is a wheel of violence and destruction with many spokes that rolls through the black community. Suicide is one of them. Others include homicides, drug addictions— including prescription drugs, as well as alcohol and tobacco use (smoking and chewing), and poor health. The same psychosocial forces contribute to all of these forms of destructive behaviors. I have constructed this wheel which shows some of the destructive behaviors that affect black people and contribute significantly to their premature deaths.

Wheel of Destructive Behaviors

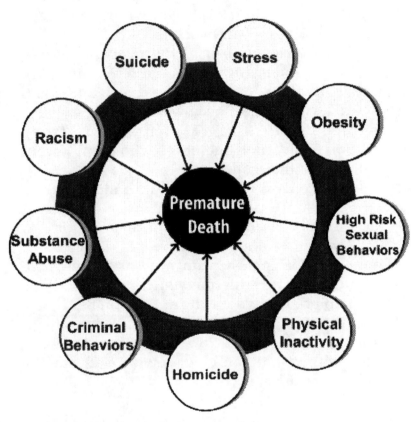

They are all interrelated and until recent years, the area of black suicide got very little attention. Finally, it is out of the closet. Black people do commit suicide and at a much higher rate than many would believe, especially among young black males ages 18 to 35.

The next section recognizes the problem of black suicide and the stories you will read show a willingness of these survivors of black suicide to share their stories with us. This process has not been easy for them. On a personal level, they have had to relive the excruciating pain and grief associated with a death by suicide. Some have also been faced with disagreements and strong opposition from family members who did not want them to share these stories.

These survivors of suicide have shared their stories in the hope that you, the reader, will understand and accept the reality that suicide is a major problem among black people. We need to become more aware and educated about what we can do to recognize the many signs and do all we can to help prevent black suicide. As you read their stories, think of how brave they are. We owe them an immeasurable debt. Now read what they have to share with you, about how they were affected by the suicide of their loved one.

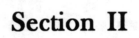

Section II

Black Survivors of Suicide—
Those Who Are Left Behind

•Surviving Dad • The Pain Of My Son's Suicide
•Why My Brother, Why? •This Is The Gun My
Husband Used To Kill Himself •Mother's Day Is
The Hardest, Since Mama Killed Herself
•My Sister! My Sister! •After 14 Years Of A
Happy Marriage, My Husband Killed Himself
•My Mother's Suicide •I Was Just A Kid When
Dad Killed Himself •An Equivocal Death:
Did He Or Didn't He.

The stories that follow are some examples of
what thousands and thousands of people experience
as survivors of suicide. They are people like you,
people like your relatives, and people like your
neighbors. They are like people you work with and
interact with in your daily activities. You may never
know the pain they deal with as survivors of suicide.
I express profound gratitude to Ain, William,
Courtney, Ruth, M.C., Bill, Crystal, Marlon, Evelyn,
and Donna. They shared their stories in the hope
that they will help heighten the awareness of suicide
as being a significant health problem that affects

thousands of black people each year—those who commit suicide and those who are affected by the deaths. I know that it is their wish that their stories will in some way contribute to the reduction of suicide among back people specifically and the reduction of suicide in general.

To those of you who contributed your stories for this book, I am acutely aware of the emotional difficulties you experienced in reliving the painful memories to present your stories for this book. I salute each of you for your courage. Thank you for your willingness to share your experiences.

Surviving Dad

The first person is Ain, who has worked tirelessly as a member of the Michigan Association for Suicide Prevention since the suicide of her father. In part, she was looking for answers, in part helping other survivors and adding to the body of knowledge about suicide prevention. Most children expect their parents to die before them but few expect them to take their own life. Ain was very close to her father and was devastated by his suicide. This is what Ain had to say:

In 2002, Dad was one of 31 people who completed suicide in the District of Columbia (DC) in that year. He hung himself with an extension cord at the age of 57. I was two months shy of 30. Thankfully, I did not find him. He was burdened by many things, past and present, in his last year of life. He ended up abandoning routine activities and withdrawing from regular contact with me and my older brother. He also surrounded himself with music and books that reinforced his negative feelings—especially material centering on the plight of black men. He died believing that he wouldn't achieve the life he wanted.

I still carry some self-blame for Dad's suicide because I never told anyone that I thought he was considering it. I actually asked him about his ideation two months before his death during a weekend visit. I was troubled by his increasingly hopeless attitude. He denied that he was suicidal, but the response bothered me. It lacked his usual indignation or sarcasm when I misjudged him. My unease remained after I returned home, so I decided to bring it up in our next conversation and then alert my family if I still felt the same. When his sister called, I knew before she said a word that I was too late and that he had killed himself. I've been able to forgive myself somewhat for how I mishandled that situation, but survivors never stop thinking that they could have saved their loved ones from themselves.

I still wish Dad had sent me one last letter. He began writing me when I started going away to school at age 14. He would usually talk about current events or detail some point he tried to make over the telephone. I usually needed a dictionary to look up some of the vocabulary he used. However, his suicide note couldn't have been more uncharacteristic. It was only a list of his demographics, perceived failures, and morbid thoughts. I didn't even take it seriously because I knew I would get a real goodbye letter when I returned home. It never came. That's when the full force of his suicide hit me. Luckily, I still have most of his letters.

I still depend on other survivors for support and insight. I was immersed in anger, self-doubt, insomnia, and answer-seeking for a year before I joined a Survivors of Suicide (SOS) support group. It wasn't easy for me to open up to complete strangers and accept their feedback. I was also warned by a former African American member not to expect many of us to attend, but I didn't care. I was desperate for help and felt immediately affirmed. SOS gave me a regular time and place to deal with my grief without stigma or the fear of burdening others. With each meeting, I still learn more about myself and how much survivor experiences can vary. I always leave with more determination to heal.

My latest effort in that regard was to write a letter of complaint to the funeral home we used, which is black-owned and based in a DC-suburb. They were fine until the day of Dad's memorial, when they forgot to give us his ashes before we left their facility and the area. Next, they reneged on their pledge to let us pick them up at our convenience. They actually presented it to me as a choice. I could either pay storage fees or receive his remains by US mail at no additional charge. But I was only given a few days to decide. I agreed to the mailing just to get him out of their hands. I still cry, remembering that encounter and delivery. Dad would have been livid!

With the letter sent, my focus now turns to correcting my anti-social tendencies. I was a shy introvert before Dad's death so my support circle had always been very small. Since the suicide, I've often limited my interactions to family and later on, SOS. It's hard to have the desire to reach out and form new friendships when I'm still wounded. I hope to make much more progress in this area during my next year of survivorship.

I also need to conquer the book. In 1997, Dad told me of an article he read about black women who were abandoned by their fathers,"Whatever Happened to Daddy's Little Girl?" written by Jonetta Rose Barras for the *Washington City Paper*. He worried that I felt forsaken when he moved from Michigan (my home) back to DC (his childhood home) in 1993. He harped on it for weeks until I convinced him that his concerns were unfounded. When I recently saw that Ms. Barras had reworked the article into a full-length book, I bought it immediately, but I haven't been able to get past the introduction. It symbolizes for me how drastically his thinking changed. I have no expectations about how I will feel afterwards, but I do think of this text as some kind of milestone and I am still compelled to surpass it.

I've started exploring suicide advocacy in my state, but I still fear that Dad's reputation will be tarnished in the process. I've been missing him a lot this year and reflecting on all the good he did for me during our 30-year history. He was not perfect, but he worked hard to defy the fatherlessness that was so publicly associated with my generation. I worry that my activities will end up putting him in a bad light. I'm also unsure if I want to "capitalize" on his death. I brought up this latter topic to an older survivor-daughter earlier this year. She said I could choose to view my work as helping others instead. I hope she's right.

My three -year journey as a survivor has been painful, exhausting, and humbling. I'm still feeling my way around and looking for better ways to live with Dad's absence. I'm far less anxious about the unexpected now and trying not to be as judgmental. It took a while to remove him from my future life vision, but his advice is never far from my mind. My worst days emerge around his death anniversaries and birthday (he would have been 60 this year). However, there are times when I can reminisce about him without even thinking about the suicide. I savor those moments whenever they arise.

Thank you, Dr. Kirk, for asking me to share my story. I also appreciate Vanessa Marie Lewis, my SOS facilitator, for her help in overcoming my writer's block. I will always be grateful to my paternal aunt, Pamela Teagle; my brother, Kofi Boone; and my best friend, Dorcas Blue Reyes for their love and concern.

The Pain of My Son's Suicide

One of the common things about parents is that we never expect to "bury our children." That is contrary to the life cycle; children usually bury their parents. However, this was not the case with the Powell family. William and Naomi are college graduates, have good, well-paying jobs and live in an upper middle class neighborhood in a suburb of Washington, D.C. They have four children. They are deeply religious, and could not have been more shocked by what happened to their son. This is what William, the father had to say:

Recently, a white co-worker sent me an email message to let me know that his son had committed suicide a few days ago. I was deeply saddened and immediately rushed down to his office to offer support and condolences. Having experienced the loss of a son, myself, I was quite familiar with the pain this could cause and I imagined that he was quite distraught and upset. When I reached his office, another gentleman he had shared the news with was also talking to him. I shook my co-worker's hand and told him I was very sorry to hear of his son's death. I departed quickly so as to avoid interfering with the conversation he was already having. What struck me, however, was the smile that he had on his face.

The next day, I sent the co-worker a brief note again offering to talk or lend support. He told me later of his son's depression illness and how he had struggled so hard over the last few years. He related a story to me about how his son asked him once, "If a person was dying from any other illness, wouldn't you rather see him out of his misery?" Therefore, it seemed my co-worker had found some measure of relief in knowing that his son was out of his misery. So, he was able to smile.

But, I was not able to smile after my son's death. For me, it was torment and pain. My story begins with June 30, 2003, a day I will never forget. It was a usual day, I thought, with work and Monday-type things. My youngest daughter, Courtney, had moved into my son's old room at the other end of the hall. My niece and other daughter, Theresa, lived at home too. All was normal. My oldest daughter, Wanda, lived in another state. Naomi, my wife, was working her usual long hours. It was strange, however, that Verizon would call at about 8PM looking for my son who had not reported to work yet. Thinking that Teet, (my son's nickname) had overslept, Theresa simply put in a call to him and said, "Hey bro. Wake up. Verizon is calling looking for you." He was supposed to be at work at 4 o'clock.

Teet had moved out about nine months prior, having been right on target for when he had planned to move out on his own. He seemed excited at the closing. I was the proudest father in the world. At 24, my son had done well. He had a good salary, a shiny, black, top-of-the-line Cherokee Jeep, and now he was moving into his own place, a condominium that was all his. He was grown now. He was so "polished" at closing, having left the thug lingo outside the door, for a while. It was amazing how he could switch from thug-talk to professional-talk with the snap of a finger. The real estate agent and the mortgage company folks at closing joined in on the pride. They were proud too, and I could tell. After all, this was something to be proud of considering what was happening with our young black men.

And Teet had even higher goals. He swore he was going to be a millionaire by age 30. And I believed him. I saw nothing standing in his way. Lately, ideas were popping out of his head left and right. I mean good, strong, solid ideas. He had an idea about setting up an internet company that completely blew my mind. He had everybody's roles laid out—me for marketing, his mother for running things, and so on. He thundered upstairs one morning after work, at 8:30 to be exact, and closed my bedroom door behind him. He said, "Pops, I got this idea!!"

I said, "What is it, son?" looking at the clock because it was time for me to get to work. Then he launched into this brilliant plan that he had constructed in his mind. I didn't understand what was going on, but it seemed he was going through some sort of metamorphosis. Man, he seemed twice as smart. His conversations were so up there. I remember asking Naomi one day, "Have you talked to your son lately?" And, when he told me he had read just about all of the "Left Behind" series, I was just in awe. I didn't even know he was reading those books.

But, all was apparently not well. Teet was hard to satisfy. The Jeep was actually his fourth automobile. He didn't like the first Honda we bought him. He didn't like the second Honda we bought him. He didn't like the sharp, silver Diamante that, this time, I let him select, himself. And, now he didn't like the Jeep. He actually wanted to trade it, but he owed more for the Jeep than he could sell it for. And, he didn't like his condo, we found out after his death. He confided to his girlfriend that he was not happy there. He hated it, she said. But, he resisted her notion to move back in with us.

Another thing that made him unhappy was that on June 30, he was supposed to start working on a new shift, a shift beginning at 4 PM. This would permit him to do things during the day that he wanted to do. But, he had to fight to get the new shift. In fact, his supervisor, whom he had complained about so much, had denied his request to move to the new shift. It was only after going through the union that he was finally able to get what he wanted so badly.

But this came with a price. Apparently, some co-workers had gotten upset about being bumped to a new shift. And the same supervisor consoled the mad workers by saying, "Blame Will. Will did it." "Will" was the name that he was known by at work.

So at 8 PM, Teet had not reported to work. And the text messages that had been a common thing between him and his girlfriend had not been taking place. By 3 AM, Tuesday morning, she convinced Courtney to wake up Naomi and me because she feared something was wrong with Teet.

On the way to his condo, I really didn't drive any faster than usual. Instinctively, I knew something awful was wrong and I was in no hurry to get there. It never occurred to me that we should have left Courtney at home. She was only 16 at the time. I can still see her wallowing on the floor screaming, "My brother is dead. My brother is dead." Naomi was down there with her. I had used a key to get in that he had given me a few months ago. He was lying on his bed, the gun still clinched in his hand, with lots on blood on the bed and floor. Somehow I managed to call the police.

The days that followed Teet's death were foggy. At first, I asked my boss not to disclose his cause of death, but I later changed my mind. The outpouring of care and concern was incredible. Cards numbered in the hundreds and flowers were everywhere. Between 600 - 800 people attended the funeral. Everyone was incredibly loving and caring.

It was surreal. We witnessed a type of love I had never witnessed before.

Things got worse after the funeral. Teet's note said he was not happy. He said he loved everyone unconditionally. He asked God to forgive him and to have mercy on his soul. But, it did not make sense that he would kill himself. We combed through everything looking for answers. It did not make sense. He was not depressed like the son of my co-worker. His girlfriend said he begged her not to leave him on Sunday, but I saw nothing wrong Saturday night when I last saw him. He popped in with a friend, used the bathroom, and left. The fact that he was gone hurt so badly. I cried every day throughout the day. Our family had been wounded. We were broken. I was broken. A self-assured, strong man was now broken, hopeless.

A couple months after the funeral, it became evident that we needed professional help to get us back to where we could function. Theresa could no longer sleep alone. We couldn't bare being alone in the house. We timed our arrivals and departures to coincide with each other. I couldn't sleep and began to break out in sweats at night. My private doctor wrote me a referral for psychiatric treatment. And, my wife made an appointment for all of us to see a local psychologist.

We went to our first counseling session around October; my memory escapes me. We went with great expectations. It was Naomi, Courtney and me that went. The girls really didn't want to go and they definitely didn't want to talk about their brother's death. The counseling was with a local clinical psychologist. She was a nice lady, at first, but she seemed a bit too professional. She asked endless questions—about our family, our son, our past, our everything. Inside, I figured she was trying to establish a cause and, secondarily, an understanding and an acceptance of Teet's death. This was probably supposed to relieve the pain. But, the process was too slow, too clinical, too detached. We did take her up on her suggestion that we attend a Suicide Support Group that met at Howard University.

The Support Group turned out to be the Survivors Circle, a support group belonging to the National Organization for People of Color Against Suicide (NOPCAS). I remember the first meeting Naomi and I attended. Our son's girlfriend was also with us. The group was supposed to go around the room and identify themselves. When it became my turn, I couldn't talk. All I could do was cry.

If my son's name had been different from mine, perhaps I would have been able to get my name out. But, his name was the same as mine and the reason for being there was too much to bear. But, Donna Barnes, the support group leader and co-founder of NOPCAS let me cry. She understood tears, because she, herself, had cried many tears over the loss of her own son to suicide. She understood the pain. She understood why Teet's girlfriend had turned to nothing but skin and bones. The other people in the group understood too. Some had lost sons, another a husband, another a mother, another a cousin. Some by hanging, some by gunshot, Donna's son by drowning. Somehow there was some strength in that weak group. The hugs of the group members were strong, and tight, and had meaning. Their faces wore expressions of understanding.

Almost three years later, Naomi and I still work with NOPCAS. We know how we benefited and we've committed to helping the organization help other people who suffer so much from the loss of a loved one to suicide. We terminated our visits to the psychologist after the second or so visit. The girls attended one or two counseling sessions but went to none of the support group meetings. It was just too painful to them.

Pulling life back together has been uphill. I can look at my son's photos now—which is a major accomplishment. Also, I just celebrated being off of sleep aids for three weeks. That too is a major accomplishment. We've even gotten a couple of hugs from Courtney lately. Through it all, our faith in God is even stronger. We believe the Lord did have mercy on our son's soul and receive him into His kingdom. Our family experiences a love deeper than anyone can imagine. Our appreciation for life and our relationship with God and mankind has taken on a brand new meaning.

♥

Why My Brother, Why?

A death by suicide has a profound affect on all members of the family. William shared how their son's death affected him as a father and as a husband. This is what his younger daughter Courtney had to say about how she was affected by the suicide of her brother. This is Courtney's story:

♥

As someone close to us passes (by going to heaven), we often ask God, "Why me and why now?" As I get older, I realize that everything happens for a reason. I may not understand it at the beginning, but eventually I try to come up with a conclusion why things happen the way they do, just so I can feel better inside.

My brother has been deceased for over three years now and it is still hard trying to grasp and understand why he had to leave me so soon. I was only sixteen years old and I felt as if my brother left me as soon as I was about to start my life and my womanhood. Not only did my brother commit suicide he brought a lot of sorrow to the family. What makes it even more difficult is that I found my own brother dead in his bed with his life drained away right before my eyes. My own sibling had taken his life away with a gun and a bullet to his brain. I never thought in a million years that my own family, my own brother, my own sibling would do such a thing to himself.

This incident was definitely a wake-up call for me and a lot of other family and friends. See, as time goes on people are getting older and life becoming harder (especially for young African Americans). My brother felt as if the only way to alleviate his pain was to kill himself, instantly, so he would feel no more pain. I can never say I understood what my brother was going through, but when you see somebody happy on the outside, it does not mean that they are happy on the inside. I think it is important to take time out of your busy schedules and spend as much time as possible with the ones you love because you never know what one is going through.

God is a superior God and I know at the end, He would never do anything that would keep me from becoming a smarter or stronger person in the long run. Live life like it is golden and never take it for granted.

The next story is about Ruth, whose husband committed suicide by using a gun. Firearms are and have been for a long time the most frequently used method of committing suicide. When I interviewed Ruth, she showed the gun to me. She had not touched it for many, many years, and it had bullets in it. This gun played a significant role in Ruth's lifelong struggle in adjusting to life without her husband. This is her story:

The year was 1981. At that time my husband, Ben, and I had been married 22 years. We had four children, one girl and three sons. Our daughter was away in college, one son was a senior in high school and the other two were living away from home.

My husband was ill with bone cancer, but he did not tell any of us. He had received a letter from the VA the weekend before he killed himself stating that there was nothing else they could do for him. Of course, he didn't show us the letter. I guess he decided then that he knew what to do.

He gave no particular indication that he was considering suicide at that time. But he always said that he would commit suicide if anything got wrong with him because he did not want anyone to have to take care of him. When he got sick, his mother and I talked about what he had said but we thought that it was just some talk he was doing because he had been sick about a year then, and he was getting progressively worse. We thought it was just his big talk, but it wasn't.

He visited his mother that day and went on out to the cemetery to his father's grave and killed himself. He was dressed the way he normally dressed and he drove his truck out there. It was on a Wednesday in December about 1:30 in the day. He left his mother's about 12:30 and went on out there. He had made up his mind before he got to his mother's house what he was going to do. He shot himself in the head.

I remember thinking after the police came to tell me, that I couldn't just fall apart, I have too many children and too much to do to fall to pieces. I had to go to the hospital to identify the body. I had to call his sister first so she could go home to be with his mother and then I had to tell his mother because I didn't want anyone from the street telling her. So I went to the hospital then rushed home so I could be there when my son got home from school.

As incredible as his death was, I was relieved that he had not killed himself at home. I could not see myself coming home and cleaning up blood before my child got home.

I wasn't really shocked when I learned of his death because my husband and I had talked about it over the years, about how he said he was going to commit suicide. He had said it so much until the way he went did not come as a complete surprise. He just didn't want to be in a position where someone would have to take care of him. He had been hospitalized several times. Things had changed quite a lot between us. For about six months before he died, he wouldn't even allow me to be alone with him in the same room. I guess he figured that he would die or something. I just don't know what he thought.

I do remember that the night before he died, we were listening to records and he was just sitting there. All of a sudden he said, "I know just what to do now."

We didn't know what he was talking about. Later, Keith and I wondered if he made up his mind at that particular point what he was going to do. But we never knew for sure.

Because he was her child, her youngest child, I asked his mother's advice in making funeral arrangements. I preferred doing what she wanted. She said she wanted him to be buried in her plot. We agreed that there would not be a wake and the funeral would be held in the funeral home chapel because he rarely spent time at the family church. His father had constructed the original church and we found out, during the funeral service that Ben had built the new church for free. None of us knew that. He never told us.

Everybody had their own way of grieving, I guess. I don't know about Tanya because the funeral was Saturday morning and her uncle who lived near the campus up there was returning that evening so he took her back. She took it okay I guess because she never appeared to have any ill effects from it. Keith, my nervous child, just changed the linen every two or three hours on all the beds just like somebody had just slept in them and he would go in, strip them and change them again. Benjamin talked a lot; he just kept talking to me, Mama so and so and so. Mama couldn't move for him. Walter, of course, was back there in the room shut up, quiet. He's quiet all the time. They all just grieved their way.

A few days after the funeral someone asked me about Ben's gun. I just happened to run into a policeman friend of mine who said he would retrieve it for me and I should come to the station on Saturday morning. When I arrived at the station, he told me it wasn't there but he promised to find it. I returned to the station a few days later and my friend told me that the gun had been sold by a policeman. He promised me that he would have the gun by Christmas Eve. When I went to the station for the gun on Christmas Eve, I was told that it was still not there. My friend told me to go home and he said, "Before this day is over the policeman who sold Ben's gun will be at your home to return it. Sure enough at a quarter to twelve, the doorbell rang and the policeman was standing there with Ben's gun and he handed it to me. He did not speak a word of greeting or apology. He just hung his head and said, "Here is your gun." He had sold it, the police officer had sold the gun. He sold it on his own and had to go and buy it back. My son, Ben, identified it. For some reason, it was very important for me to get that gun back.

I still have the gun. I don't know what to do with it but I still have it. I wouldn't have a clue how to shoot it, but I still have it. It is a sorrowful memento.

♥

My Mother's Suicide

There was a time when people in general and black people specifically believed that mental disorders like depression did not affect black people. This is obviously not true. The following story is that of a young woman whose mother died by suicide after many years of suffering from bipolar depression.

This story also shows how important it is to seek appropriate professional help to deal with a loved one's suicide. M.C. sought both individual therapy as well as help from Survivors of Suicide Group (SOS). This is her story:

Sunday, October 27, 2002 changed my life forever. I received a devastating phone call on the morning of the 27th from the person whom I aspired to be like, my mother. She apologized for not being able to live life anymore. She said that she had to take herself out. At the age of 23 years old, it was the most painful experience for me to hear my mother tell me that she wanted to take her own life. Her suicide was the result of a ten-year battle with a severe mental illness, bipolar disorder.

From my life as an adolescent to a young adult, I saw my mother excel professionally as a French professor, a Fulbright Scholar, and a docent at The Smithsonian National Museum of African Art. Toward the end of her life I saw her decline into a severe depression with the inability to get out of bed for days at a time. There were several admittances to the psychiatric ward at our local hospital. She also experienced excessive weight gain, a marital separation, unemployment, filing for bankruptcy, and she ended her life with the loss of hope. Seeing such a variation in my mother's life left me confused and unable to understand why all of this was happening.

My mother had previously made a suicide attempt. This effort will always stay fresh in my mind. About a year before her suicide, my brother and I found her in our garage with the car running. We had to open the car door and drag her out of the car and back into the house. My father took her to the hospital. She was admitted to the psychiatric ward for two weeks. I can remember being so thankful that we were able to stop her from ending her life. Never would I have thought that she would be successful in her attempt. We later found out that she had stopped taking her medication for the bipolar disorder. Every time she was feeling better she would stop taking her medication, which would make her slump into a deep depression.

My mother's suicide left me with a lot of different emotions. After being called into a room by the doctor and being told that she had gone into cardiac arrest, I immediately felt like a helpless child who had been abandoned by her mother. I could not comprehend how I was supposed to go on with my life without the person who supported me the most emotionally and to whom I looked up to. This was the first time that I had experienced such pain. It felt like a void had been left that was so deep in my heart that it could never be filled. I was very angry with my mother and could not believe how she had left my brother and me so suddenly. I felt like, how dare she end her life and not be able to share the milestones in my brother's and my life like his graduating from high school and going to college and my one day getting married and having children.

Along with the abandonment and anger, I felt a lot of guilt. The day before my mother's death, she had invited me to go to lunch with her. I refused to go, because at the time I did not understand her illness. I told her that I did not want to be seen in public with her, because she had really let her appearance go. The last year of her life she looked very depressed and hopeless. It was hurtful to not have my mother look as she did in my adolescent and teenage years, happy and positive about life.

Immediately following my mother's death, I wanted to die too. I was left behind and confused as to why I should continue to live life. Each night I prayed that the Lord would take me too. During my commute to work I would look at the train tracks and wonder what it would be like if I stepped out into the path of an oncoming train.

With the inability to know how to bear all of the pain of losing my mother, I knew that I needed professional help. I sought the assistance of a grief counseling center, the William Wendt Center in Washington, DC, a couple of weeks after her death. I started going to individual therapy once a week and a suicide survivors support group twice a month. I went to individual therapy for a year and a half and I attended the support group for three years. I truly believe they both saved my life. The support group helped me to know that I wasn't the only one going through this. It was a safe place to share my pain with people who could understand me. I met many people who were going through or had experienced the same feelings from their loved one's suicide. I was also able to meet other young adults whose parent had committed suicide.

Both experiences were extremely beneficial to me because it was hard to talk to my family about what had happened. My friends were very supportive and were willing to listen, but did not understand the extent of my pain. Most of my family does not talk about my mother's suicide. It is like the elephant in the room for them. The suicide is there, but no one wants to talk about it. Some members of my extended family are not even aware that my mother committed suicide. They were told that my mother had an illness that she was suffering with and died suddenly. It is as if she died a shameful death.

My mother suffered with a mental illness. Mental illness runs in her family, but it is never talked about. Some of her nieces, nephews, cousins, aunts, and uncles have a severe mental illness, but are not supported, because some members of our family do not believe in mental illness. Others believe that it is not hereditary; it is something that is self-inflicted. My family's response to my mother's suicide has helped me to realize that it is imperative that a person with a mental illness receives support from his or her family. Since the loss of my mother, holidays have been very difficult for me. Thanksgiving and Christmas used to be my favorite holidays. They are now my least favorite holidays, because my mother is not here to enjoy them with me.

Mother's Day is the hardest holiday for me. I used to take my mother out to dinner each year. Now I dread each Mother's Day. For the weeks leading up to the holiday there are reminders on the radio, television, and in stores about getting a present to honor your mother on her special day. From mid-April to Mother's Day I try my best to avoid any such advertisements. I always think to myself, what are you supposed to do if your mother is no longer with you? I selfishly become angry with all of the people who still have their mothers and ask God, "Why did it have to be mine?"

I strongly believe that everything happens for a reason and have decided to use the traumatic experience of my mother's suicide to help others suffering with a mental illness. Since August 2003 I have been volunteering at a non-profit organization that provides community living for women with a mental illness. I feel that since I wasn't able to help my mother it is my mission to help these women.

My Sister, My Sister

There is always a degree of shame, confusion and embarrassment associated with suicide. Bill was one of my college roommates and a friend whom I had known since 1957. It was not until 1999, while attending the annual conference of American Association of Suicidology in New York City where Bill lived that I learned that he had lost a sister to suicide in the early 1970s. This is what Bill had to say:

Suicide is something you never forget and you never expect it to happen to your family. I remember the day as if it was yesterday. March 19, 1971. I was watching the NVAA tournament and Fordham was playing. When the call came, I did not want to believe it. My father and I had to go to Connecticut to identify the body; I could not do it. My sister once told me she did not want to live past 30 years. She was 31. The only things that kept her alive that long were her children; she had three daughters. Two were from marriage and one from a fellow (Italian) whom she lived with after her separation her husband.

My mother died when I was two and my sister was four. I was the only boy and the youngest. My mother died from childbirth and I later found out they had to drive to Greensboro to a black hospital, which complicated matters. It was tough but my father kept us together until we were teenagers and my oldest sister graduated from high school and went to New York. My sister Helen was very beautiful and everyone made over her and wanted to adopt her. She resented being the pretty one and I think my sister disliked her for getting a lot of attention. We were only two years apart and very close. My sister was not as good in school as I was and did not receive respectable grades. She ran away from home a couple of times. My father and I would go looking for her; the longest stint was about a year, she went to High Point, N.C. and returned for her senior year in high school.

She always had a lot of suitors; I was really her chaperone on dates. The one thing I noticed was that she never really seemed happy in a relationship; she told me she never felt truly loved. She had one boy friend that she seemed to like but he did not receive the approval of the family and was not allowed to come to the house. She later told me that she really liked him. She eventually got pregnant during her senior year and marched down the aisle seven months pregnant. This caused a lot of problems because the father was a H. S. star and his family objected to the relationship and his fatherhood. After graduation, my sister went to live with relatives in Detroit and her future husband went into the Marines. He came out of the Marines and they got married and went to New Haven, Connecticut where his father lived and they settled there and had another daughter.

Things seemed to be going fine. I graduated from college and settled in New York with my sister. We would visit often and things seemed fine. Then I noticed some changes; my sister went through states of depression. There were lots of quarrels and finally my sister was admitted to a state hospital for periods of time. Each time it seemed to get worse, she seemed so confused and could not cope with her surroundings. She and her husband separated and she took the girls. Her husband was a very good provided and never tried to take the girls. She met a young fellow in the institution and got pregnant. She eventually moved to New York City. I tried to help but she was sicker than I realized. The young man was just as unstable as she was and the whole family and myself were upset with the relationship. After the baby was born, she moved back to Connecticut. We talked a lot but I was distant due to the relationship because they fought physically and I wanted to kill him.

I knew things were getting out of hand but I also felt helpless. I do not know if drugs, other than prescription, were involved. My sister was in and out of the state hospital and her depression worsened. At first it was hard for me to accept her suicide because I blamed her lover. But she shot herself at close range through the head. There was no note and only her youngest daughter was present.

We fought for custody of her daughter and lost. Her boyfriend committed suicide about four years later. Seeing him at the funeral and trial really brought out the anger. It took me about two years to get over the ordeal. All of her daughters are grown and I see them quite often. I took the youngest down South to meet her black relatives. She is a beautiful girl and reminds me so much of her mother.

My sisters were very hurt by the ordeal. My sister who lives in Harrisburg led the custody fight. My oldest sister was an alcohol abuser during the time and had a lot of problems of her own. My father was very strong and came up and stayed with my sister when she lived in New York City. He died of cancer about five years after my sister's death. Now you can see why I never married.

I do not think that I have put a closure to my sister's suicide. It was really hard at first. It was so hard at first because of how she herself and the fellow she was living with, there was physical abuse, and they were constantly fighting. I asked if she wanted to come and live with me, but I knew she would never do that. Then there was the fight for the custody of her youngest daughter. Every time I went to that courtroom, I wanted to kill him. After my sister's funeral, we took her daughter to live with my sister in Harrisburg. He kidnapped her and brought her back to New Haven and we lost the custody battle. In a way, it worked out with her being around her sisters. Her grandmother raised her. We were allowed visiting rights and she is now 26 years old and we are close. I tried to catch her up with the Motley side of her family. She and her sisters get along like sisters. We have family get-togethers at Christmas and Thanksgiving. I regret that she had to grow up at such a low economical level.

The girls really help me to put closure to my sister's death because I see so much of her in each one of them.

When it first happened, I really had a hard time getting my life back together. I turned to the church. It was not enough for me. It was bad for me too because I lost my job with CBS due to a cutback, my whole world turned upside down. She was the only sister that I was close to and my sister in New York was hitting rock bottom with her drinking.

I cannot remember exactly what changed, but through the seventies, I had it rough, working grant-funded jobs and getting involved coaching basketball. I also l played football on a semi-pro team and found out that I was a good football player. The team eventually became the best semi-pro in the country. I injured my knee in an all-star game on Astro-Turf. I still have a limp from that injury. That is when I got heavily involved in coaching. I went to the "Y" to rehab and ended up running the basketball program. I am considered one of the top amateur coaches in the N.T.C.

I also realized that my science degree would not help me in the field I had chosen, so I went to Fordham to get my Master's. Still working on the PhD.

The one thing that helped me, learning more about mental illness and understanding that it is an illness and must be treated that way. Growing up, I did not know how to cope and what mental illness was all about. People who were mentally sick, we considered "crazy." More understanding and knowledge and people like you enlightening us. There was a time when black people did not commit suicide.

You know, it's fun, when you are poor and less knowledgeable and you are not stressed with mental problems. With the big bucks, here come the problems.

I think by my involvement with sports, doing something I really like and going back to school helped me to put closure to the tragedy of my sister's suicide. When her youngest daughter and I became friends, that really put closure to her death. She looks more like my sister than any of the other two.

When you feel good about your life and your accomplishments, it makes it all worth the fight, Kirk. I am not very spiritual; I'm too much of a realist. I wanted my sister back, but deep down I knew she did not want to be here and let her go. Earlier, my dreams were about her. It was like every night movie, I relived my life with my sister. I loved her very much; I still miss her and always will.

It Changed My Life Forever

Crystal is a remarkable woman who has endured a great deal since the suicide death of her husband Robert. They had two sons and were living a good life until she lost her spouse by suicide. This is Crystal's story:

"I had been happily married for fourteen years to the most wonderful man in the world. We had two great sons Mark, thirteen and Marlon, eight.

My husband had served in the U. S. Marine Corps. Robert was always a hard worker; he was very dependable and served unofficially as an advisor to many of his co-workers at the Department of Corrections where he had worked for fourteen years. People would often telephone him at home at all kinds of hours to discuss a problem or seek his advice. I sometimes felt that this interfered with our family time. When I would bring it up, he'd say that they needed him. He was a captain and took his job seriously. At times I felt too much so. Other than this type of thing, we had no real serious marital or family problems.

I'll never forget the morning of January 22, 1990. It had snowed and the ground was covered. Robert had left the house; I thought he was going to the store for something. I looked out the kitchen window and saw fooprints gong to the garage. I noticed that the garage door was still down. There were no car tracks indicating that the car had been driven out the garage. I told Mark to go to the garage to see what his dad was doing. Then I went into the bedroom, saw his drawer where he kept his gun was open. It was not there.

Just then Mark ran into the house crying and screaming, "Dad is hurt." I ran outside to the garage. I saw Robert lying there, blood around his head. I ran back into the house and called 911. Then I called my mom and told her that Robert had shot himself. The paramedics arrived and they administered first aid and took him to the hospital. By this time all the neighbors were out asking questions, being nosy. My mom arrived shortly after I called her. I think she took me to the hospital.

Robert never regained consciousness; he died the next day, January 23, 1990 at 9:50 pm.

My emotions were confused; I had all kinds of feelings. I was hurt, angry, confused, scared and embarrassed. The police questioned me. There was an investigation which I learned was typical in the case of a death. Robert's employer and co-workers were questioned also.

Robert had been depressed and stressed due to the nature of his work in the prison. He was being seen by a doctor and was taking several medications that had been prescribed for him including one for depression. There were all kinds of rumors and gossip concerning Robert's death. Everything from me shooting Robert, that he was a drug dealer, that he was involved with another woman, that I was involved with another man. It was a horrible experience; not only did I have to deal with the suicide death of my husband but all of this other bullshit.

I later learned that when Mark went to the garage he heard what he described as a growling sound; he thought that his father had bought a puppy. When he went to the front of the car he saw his father lying there bleeding and making strange sounds. That's when he ran in the house and told me that his dad was hurt. His father had shot himself in the right temple with his personal weapon, a 38. This experience was very hard on Mark.

After several weeks of police investigation, depositions and all the rumors and gossip that surrounded my husband's death, I was sick and tired of all the mess. While I loved my husband, I was angry with him for what he had done. How

could he do this to me? How could he leave his
children? I just couldn't understand it. In order to
get away from this horrible situation, and most of
all, to protect my children, I moved to another town.
I wanted and needed a new start for me and my
boys.

Both my boys and I spent time in
psychotherapy. We had several therapists—a white
female, a white male and eventually we saw a black
male psychotherapist who had some experience in
black suicide. Even though he lived in a city many
miles away, I was willing to make the drive for the
sake of my sons. He was helpful but no person or
no amount of psychotherapy can help me completely
forget or remove the pain caused by the suicide
death of my husband, the father of our children.

We are now grandparents and I often think of
Robert and how he missed the boys growing up
and seeing our granddaughters. No one will ever be
able to take the place of Robert.

I Was Just A Kid

Marlon is the younger of Robert's two sons. He
was eight years old when his father committed
suicide. This is what Marlon had to say:

I remember my dad as being a quiet man. I
know that he worked late. I loved my dad. I
remember people talking about me when my dad
died. They said that I would not understand what
my dad had done; they said I was too young to

understand and that I would not remember what happened. After all, I was just a kid. I was just a kid but I remember the crying, I remember the noise, I remember all the people, the policemen, the ambulance people, the neighbors, and the relatives. I remember being angry with my dad for killing himself. As I look back, I became very mean and controlling after his death. I remember relatives; especially my uncles telling me you got to be a man now. I didn't know what they meant by that.

I know that the word *suicide* always causes me to feel something inside.   As I was growing up, whenever someone talked about suicide—especially in a joking way—I would ask him or her to stop, not to do that. When I was in the twelfth grade, one of my friends committed suicide. I was sad, hurt and angry all over again.

My dad's suicide changed my life. I don't know what my life would have been like if he had lived, but I do know that it would have been better for me, my brother and my mom, especially my mom, had he not killed himself.

A Case of Equivocal Suicide

"I know in my heart that my husband did not commit suicide."

The official classifications of death are natural, accidental, suicide or homicidal or undetermined. The following vignette is an example of what is known as an equivocal suicide. one in which the classification of death is unclear. As you read the following pages you will see that Evelyn, this mother, this now-widow believes that her husband's death was a homicide, not a suicide. However, it was officially listed as a suicide death. This is Evelyn's story:

Having watched my lovely daughter, Dawn, receive a degree in psychology just three months prior and retiring from my job as a media specialist after thirty-two years, I was ready to enjoy life to its fullest. I was finally going to do some of the things I wanted to do but never had the time.

All my plans went awry on August 5, 1994. Since I retired from working, I boasted of having retired from the kitchen, too. We ate out quite a lot. It had been some time since my family had enjoyed what we considered a country dinner, especially one cooked by me. I thought I would surprise them, so I cooked a dinner of fresh green cabbage, meat loaf, potatoes, hush puppies and iced tea. Just as usual, my husband, Doug, called home around 6 p.m. to ask what we were eating. He laughed when I told him what dinner was and said he'd planned to take us out to eat, but he was on his way home immediately if I had cooked. We ate around 6:30 and he talked of how good the food was as he went back for seconds. The rest of the evening we laughed, talked and watched television as usual.

Around 11:15, my daughter's friend came by the house. He worked a shift that ended at 11 p.m. and the job is about fifteen minutes from the house. When he entered the house, Dawn immediately told him I'd cooked cabbage, meat loaf, and potatoes. Doug said that it was really good and that Dawn should warm some for him.

When they proceeded to the kitchen, he said he needed to go to the car lot in Bailey to pick up a car that needed some repairs to take to the main car lot in Wilson, where he worked. Since the main car lot was closer to us, he indicated that if he picked the car up tonight, then he could go directly there in the morning without having to go all the way across town. This made sense to me so I had no reason to doubt that this was the case.

About 15 or 20 minutes after he left he called back to say he was going to ride around for a while and perhaps drink a beer. When I asked him why, for he was not in the habit of drinking beer, he told me had just had a bad day. I asked him what brought this on. He said he didn't know, but he would be home in a little while. I decided I would stay up so I could find out just what was going on. But he never came back.

Early the next morning I went to the car lot to see if he had stayed there for the night, but he was not there. I called the car lot in Bailey and he had not been there either. After driving around for a while to places I felt he could possibly be, I came back home and called a friend at the police department.

A special detective was put on the case to look for him. Calls were made to friends and family outside the state but to no avail. Neighbors took it upon themselves to look for him. The car lot where he worked and the surrounding area was the first place they looked. I personally asked the detective to search the car lot. He sent a canine unit to search and informed me that nothing was to be found. Approximately three days later, the car he was driving was spotted just in back of the car lot and he was found inside, the victim of apparent suicide. My neighbors who had been looking for him said, no, this cannot be for we already looked here. A note was found that was written to his mother, sister-in-law, and me that said in addition to some other things "you'll never be able to understand this so don't try."

There was never a thorough investigation. I had to request an autopsy through the state medical examiner. The local medical examiner would not grant one. The death scene was never secured. I was able to walk straight to the car on the day he was found. The state medical examiner was led to believe it was a clear cut case of suicide so she never checked for any drugs or anything else in the body. My husband was not a drinker. He had rarely had a drink in the last fifteen to twenty years. He would drink a beer on occasion with special friends. He had not had a beer to my knowledge within the past year or two. Having been married to this man for 30 years, I noticed no signs indicating that something was going on in his life that would cause him to commit suicide.

I had a conference with the detective who was on the case and the interim police chief concerning the ordeal and told them of my suspicions. They indicated to me that they had reason to believe that he was seeing some young lady and that might be the reason for his suicide. This to me didn't make sense. I checked with the physician to see if there was any medical reason why he would commit suicide; there was none. Not being satisfied, I sought help from the newly appointed police chief some three or four months later so that I might find some closure. He graciously said yes he would look into the matter. After a few days, he called to say that there was nothing in the file except the autopsy report and I had a copy of that. There were no names of people who had been questioned. Consequently, he was at a loss to help me because of lack of information. His apology for such a 'shoddy job' did not help my peace of mind in the least.

Since those times I've had people tell me that Doug's boss was one of the biggest drug dealers in the country. And that there had been other incidents of his employees being beaten and killed. I do know that his only correspondence to me consisted of the statement, "Mrs. Hagans, we are going to pursue this death. I don't believe Doug killed himself." He never came to visit nor did he attend the funeral. My only fact-to-face dealings with him came when I initiated a visit after the funeral was over.

It's been two years since my husband's death and I miss him more and more each day. It seems funny that I miss him more on Saturday and Sunday than any other day during the week. I somehow feel that it's because we spent more time together on these two days. Our weekends started on Saturday around 2 p.m. I always looked forward to his coming home so that we could get in the car and just ride around to places where he was born or grew up. Many times we ventured to Winterville, where I was born, and surrounding towns. He would tease me about the town with one stoplight. We would laugh, tease and enjoy each other's company; just the two of us. We knew where the best restaurants were within one hundred miles from home. We must have eaten in most of them. Doug was adventurous and liked to try different things. He would always take a different route to places we visited so he could see how many ways there were to get there. Sometimes it would be midnight or 1 a.m. Sunday morning when we'd finally get home.

Then came Sunday, always church and afterwards Sunday dinner. Whether it was out or at home, we always ended up sitting down on Sunday afternoon to watch football, basketball or a great western movie. We liked most of the same things. This doesn't seem like a lot but it meant a lot to me just to have someone to be with, to talk to, to laugh with. Now, many times I find myself angry! I ask myself why me. I hate to see holidays come, especially Christmas. Doug loved Christmas like a little kid. Our wedding anniversary and birthdays are totally disastrous. All I've ever wanted was to be happy and to make someone else happy in the process. I never go the places we used to go together. The friends we shared as a couple have seemingly forgotten that we were friends. When other widows told me this would happen, I said, 'not my friends.' Believe me, it's true. I get no invitations to many of the things I used to get invited to.

There is consolation in knowing that I serve a God who I feel will one day reveal to me just what really happened. While it may not be all that I want to know, I feel sure it will be all that I need to know. Many times during the past two years, I have faced the problem of what I would do 'if.'

Financially, I am fine. The fear came when I had problems with my car. I never knew what it meant to worry about having a flat tire. Does the oil need changing? What does the mechanic mean when he says your 'rack and pinion' is bad? Is he taking advantage of me because I am a woman? It's snowing, who can I call to take me to the store? What gentleman can I call without worrying if his wife will mind? Many times I am lonely. I need someone to talk to, someone to go out with. It's been real easy to say, this would not have been if Doug were here.

Dawn is a quiet young woman who feels that she must solve all the world's problems. Certainly you are familiar with the statement 'A little learning is a dangerous thing'. She spent four years at NCCU and majored in psychology and feels that she has the answer to it all. While she grieves, it is in a way that the average person would not recognize, but I'm her mother. There are times when she goes into a shell, is very quiet and ceases to say much to me. She was always a 'father's child'. If she got sick during the night, it was daddy that she called first. Now she has no one to call. Around special days, she tends to get sick or so she would have me believe. I know now that it is during these times when she misses her dad most and she grieves. I've learned that she says that she is sick so as not to have me know that she is grieving. While she visits my family very easily and constantly calls them, Doug's family is a different story. She will not visit or call them unless I insist. It brings back too many memories. Her greatest fear is what she will do when she marries. Who will walk her down the aisle? After a long conversation about this, we've finally decided that several men will get the pleasure of walking her down the aisle. They will be her father's best friends who have remained that way since his death. She will place them strategically down the aisle and each will escort her to the other. If they cease to remain true friends, she will walk alone with her father's memory.

As I said, I get angry many times. When I was able to get my daughter to finally talk to me about how she felt and this conversation evolved, I became even angrier. I thought how dare someone deprive my child of the right to have her father escort her down the aisle. Even though marriage was not in sight, I began immediately to find a solution to the problem for my one and only child.

Closure is not easy because there are so many people I come in contact with who were special to Doug and vice versus. My optometrist told me that he cannot stand to go past the car lot that Doug ran because he liked Doug so much. Doug called this man, "My white brother." My medical doctor always talks about the fact that when I was being treated for breast cancer, Doug never let me go to the doctor alone. He was always with me even though I was perfectly capable of driving myself. Whenever I go for checkups, I am always emotional because I remember. You might say I could change doctors, I can't. I love the man who helped me get through my ordeal. He was more than a doctor to me, he was also my friend. Yet, every time I see him, I remember. It seems that everywhere I turn, I am reminded.

I am not trying to forget Doug, just the senselessness of his death. It does get better. I am sure closure will be more evident when I find that gentleman who can take me out to eat, call me on the phone, spend a few hours at my house or me at his, say those things a woman likes to hear. In other words, I need to feel like a needed woman again. I've never ceased to feel like a woman, but not a needed woman; there is a difference. I still have desires just to be held and talked to. It is a woman thing.

Dawn has moved to Charlotte, North Carolina. She has renewed acquaintances with a young man who has always loved and respected her. They are dong fine. She loves her job working with abused youth and youth offenders. She still thinks she is supposed to solve all the world's problems. Somehow, I feel that she might one day be a child psychologist. Wouldn't that be something?

Meanwhile we weather our storms by showering each other with more love and affection than we did before Doug's death, if that is possible. We've learned that it's all right to let each other know how we feel. I realize that it is all right for her to know that there are still times in my life when it all comes back as fresh as new and I still cry. She finds comfort in decorating his grave for Christmas and putting several presents under the tree for me just as he did. I make sure that she is remembered on all the occasions that she was remembered when her dad was alive and then some.

If any good has come out of his untimely death, I guess it's the fact I didn't have to go back to work after having retired. The part-time job I do was something I planned before his death and it is truly a means of getting out of the house and meeting people. As morbid as a job at the funeral home may sound, it helps me because I get to help others.

Mother's Loss

People respond to suicide of a loved one in a variety of ways. They range from denial that the death was a suicide to never talking about that person or the death, especially outside of the family circle. Donna did something very remarkable, she not only talked about the suicide of her son Marc publicly, but she also, with several others who had lost children to suicide, started the first National Organization for People of Color Against Suicide (NOPCAS). The first and only organization created specifically to focus on suicide education and prevention among black people and people of color. Donna is the president and executive director of NOPCAS. This is her story:

November 6, 1990

I was lying on the couch, probably smoking a cigarette and watching TV, when the phone rang. I glanced at the clock on the VCR that read 10:29 p.m. I picked up the phone and said, "Hello."

The voice on the other end said, "Mrs. Barnes, this is Dr. McLean at the University of Lowell. I am calling to let you know that I was informed that your son left his dorm room around 7:30 this evening. It appears that he left some notes to his roommate that may be considered suicide notes."

My knees buckled. I really never understood what that meant until that night. I almost fell, but held on to the table. My mind quickly went to the last time I had spoken to Marc which was three days before. He seemed okay, had something to tell me about what his advisor said to him, but couldn't talk because his roommate was in the room. And for the past three days, I had been trying to reach him to find out what it was.

Marc had apparently left his dorm, but was not found until seven months later. During that time the family and I, with the assistance of a national missing person's organization, conducted a massive search to no avail.

May 28, 1991

Around 2:30 p.m. in the afternoon, a local policeman knocked on my door. "Ma'am," he said, as handed me a piece of paper, "please call this number."

I asked why and what was wrong. He said my car was found. I told him my car was right there in the driveway; he must be making a mistake. He asked if I had reported a brown 1979 Camaro missing. I got extremely excited and said, "Yes, yes....they must have my son!" and ran into the house to make the phone call. I was anxious to talk to my son. I had so much to tell him and so many questions to ask.

"Hi, this is Donna Barnes. I was told to call this number. How are you?"

The voice on the other end said, "Yes, ma'am; I am doing fine and I am sorry to tell you that your son's car has been found at the bottom of the Merrimack River."

I responded with something positive because I was thinking there might have been a clue as to where he was.

"Ma'am, I am sorry to say that his body was found in the car."

I thought to myself, *the search is finally over. Now we have our answer.* And began feeling numb. I peeked into the living room at my 16-year-old daughter who was contentedly watching a talk show, then said, "Thank you," to the voice on the other end and hung up.

The Merrimack River, where the car was found, was two blocks from his dorm. Marc's car had simply begun to rise up from the water because they were lowering the level of the river that day. They did it every spring and every summer; heavy objects come to the surface. The search was over and it was apparent that my son most likely drove his car into the Merrimack River on purpose. The speedometer read 40 miles an hour. There was no alcohol in his system, no drugs. Sometimes, like Julius Erving (whose son's body was found in his car at the bottom of a pond), I would like to believe it was an accident, but the notes he left behind kept me from doing that.

December 4, 1994 – A Safe Place, Somerville, MA

- My name is Larry. Sheila, my live-in mate, committed suicide eight years ago.
- My name is Joan. My brother, Jerry, killed himself in 1987.
- My name is Lucinda. My son, William, took his life seven years ago.
- My name is Sarah. My son, Richard, committed suicide five months ago.
- I'm Gerald, Richard's father.
- My name is Susan. I have two friends who committed suicide three years ago.
- My name is Patricia. My son, Samuel, committed suicide two years ago.
- My name is Jean. My mother killed herself nine years ago and my sister, Sidney, killed herself a few months ago.
- My name is Sally. My daughter, Jennifer, committed suicide in July.

- My name is Linda. I am Jennifer's aunt.
- My name is Bill. My son, Conrad, killed himself last year.
- My name is Ruth. I am Conrad's mother.
- My name is Donna. My son, Marc, took his life four years ago.

A Safe Place was started in 1978 by a woman and her husband who wanted to share their grief over the loss of their daughter with other suicide survivors. No matter where they turned, they could not find enough room for their grief during the year after their daughter killed herself by jumping from the roof of a five-story building in Newbury, Massachusetts.

One night, as the story goes, not quite six months after their daughter's death, the couple was at a relative's house for dinner. The wife had been warned by friends and relatives that it usually takes six months to get over the death of a loved one, and that people would expect her to "shape up her act." However, she was still wrestling with the thought of it all and reeling with grief. That night, at dinner, she began talking about her daughter's suicide. Suddenly, her brother-in-law interrupted. "Knock it off," he said, "enough is enough."

The woman was mortified but forced a smile and said, "Wait, it's only five and a half months – I still have two weeks!"

It took me four long years to join this support group. The most compelling need I had after we finally buried my son and said good-bye was the when and why? The answers to suicide are not easily obtained. All the information surrounding the event was needed in an effort to put the pieces together.

I was confused. My mind was reeling with questions: *When did he die? Was it the day he was reported missing from his dorm room? Or did he drive around for a few days, weeks, months...contemplating. Why did he get $10 from the ATM that night as was indicated in his bank record? Why did he have $28 on him when his body was found? If he had $18, why did he need $10 more? Marc very seldom had money on him. Why did he take his life when he had a loving family, had friends at home and at school, had a good conversation with my mother the week before to wish her a happy birthday. He also spoke with his cousin to say hi and told me with great joy that he spoke with Brian at Nana's house. He called his girlfriend a few days before to let her know he would see her in a few weeks during the Thanksgiving weekend. He put his car in the shop and paid $175 to get it out just a couple of days before. What was going on in his head? What was I missing? He didn't appear to be someone who was going through despondency. He wasn't giving up. He was making plans.*

Creating an Organization Called NOPCAS

A writer from the Boston *Globe*, Francis Latoure, wanted to do a front-page story on suicide among African Americans. She was doing her homework and noticed several articles in the archives on Marc when he was missing and when his body was found. She wanted to interview a parent who had lost someone to suicide and was glad to learn there was someone right in her back yard.

She gave me a call to set up an interview and was intrigued about the work that I was already doing in the area of suicide among African Americans and decided to include a sizeable picture of me in the article with contact information. That article was the beginning of my professional career in suicidology in terms of community involvement. The article came out on April 27, 1997. That Sunday morning when I got the newspaper, I read the article and decided to call my family to let them know about it. Most were supportive while some wondered why I would spill my guts out for all to read. I did feel a little exposed and uneasy, but also felt like this article was doing something, but I was not quite sure what. I only hoped that it was worth disclosing my son's suicide.

That Monday morning I showed up to my office at Northeastern University. Only a chosen few knew I had lost a son to suicide, others just knew that suicide was my area of concentration and probably felt my interest stemmed from perhaps being suicidal...or attempting suicide. No one ever asked me about my interest. That Monday, people came up to me and said how surprised they were that I had lost a son. One woman was actually upset with me because she thought we were close and couldn't understand why I had never told her.

Another said to me, "But you always have this smile on your face."

And another did not know what to say so she just said, "Are you okay?"

The men had no comment, just said simply, "nice article." However, one male colleague posted the whole article on the door to the mailroom.

What I did not know was that on that same day, Daniel Augustine Pimienta III hanged himself in the basement of his family home in Teaneck, New Jersey. When his mother went to her mailbox the following day, she found the article that someone left in her mailbox. She could not read it then and just put it aside. In the fall of 1997, Lois Talisferro, Daniel's mother finally read the article left in her mailbox and decided to give me a call.

We had several conversations, but it wasn't until November of that year that she insisted that something needed to be done. She called me after Thanksgiving to inform me that on Thanksgiving Day her anxiety caused her to break the dining room table in half. She was upset, she was angry and *wham*. She also mentioned that there were several other suicides in Teaneck's black community and couldn't understand what was going on. "We need to do something," she cried.

I asked if she wanted me to come to her. She responded positively and thought that maybe I could speak to the other families about suicide. I said, "When?"

She said, "Anytime."

I said, "How about February?"

She said, "Okay."

I knew this was something I could not do on my own and that I needed to team up with some other survivors. I called a woman I met in Atlanta, Doris Smith, to see if she would go with me and she said she could. I called Les Franklin, who had lost his son, Shaka, in 1990 to suicide. Les had been on the Phil Donahue Show and was interviewed for the Boston *Globe* article. He also responded favorably and said to let him know the details.

I thought to myself, *okay, we are going to Teaneck to talk to a few folks about losing their loved one to suicide. We need a venue.* I called Karen Dunne-Maxim, whom I had met at several conferences. In my conversation with her, she always felt I needed to meet other black survivors because she had a gut feeling we needed to unite. I told her my plan and she was ecstatic. She said she would find some to make this happen, and she did. I contracted with a hotel in Teaneck for a meeting room. I asked for a small one because we figured about ten people would be there. Doris, Les, and I met at the hotel one evening, had dinner and talked in to the wee hours of the night. We had a lot to share about our experiences.

The next day, Karen arranged for us to do a panel discussion at her place of employment and invited about 15 people. We went back to the hotel and set up for our meeting the following day. We arrived at the meeting room and were surprised to see seating for about 25 people. We knew there were four families who lost someone to suicide and figured one or two family members from each family would attend. What we did not know was that Lois had gone to the local newspaper to tell them we were coming to town.

On the front page of the local Teaneck newspaper was a picture of Lois holding Danny's military picture with a caption, *Blacks confront the pain of suicide. Surviving parents break silence on a problem often hidden among minorities.* The meeting entitled "Sharing the Pain," was announced with the time, date, and location.

That Saturday morning, I strolled down to the lobby level of the hotel on my way to the meeting room. My daughter had come to help out and was already downstairs at the registration desk. There was a line. I walked past the desk and into the meeting room. Almost every seat was taken. I looked at my watch and it was 8:45 a.m. The meeting was scheduled to start at 9 a.m. People were there on time and waiting. I quickly called catering and asked for more box lunches to be added to our small order. At 8:55, Doris, Les, and I walked to the front of the room and took a seat behind the head table. We looked out at the crowd and saw standing room only. We asked everyone to introduce themselves and found that not only parents of loved ones lost to suicide, but also lawyers, guidance counselors, teachers, mental health providers, and the funeral director were in attendance.

We realized these people were there for answers. We each told our story and more. By noon we told everyone they could step outside to take a lunch break, since box lunches had been set up in the foyer. Several people asked if would be okay to get their box lunch and bring it back into the room so that they could continue the meeting. And that's what happened. We grabbed a lunch, took our seats back at the table, and chewed our food while one of us talked.

There was good discussion coming from the audience, too. People were making testimonies, people were making suggestions on what was needed in our communities, and people were listening intensively. By 5 p.m. it was down to 20 attendees.

All were survivors, and all found it hard to leave. I am not sure what it is about meeting with other survivors for the first time after experiencing a loss, but I could honestly relate to those who lingered.

My very first support group meeting four years after Marc's death was in Somerville, Massachusetts in the evening. When the meeting ended, I did not want to leave. I stayed there chatting with others who did not want to leave. It was tough. This is what happens at the first meeting with other survivors (whether it is a support group or professional meeting): you feel comfortable within the group . . .warmth. . . a safety zone. . . no one will hurt you or say insensitive things. . . no one will judge you for losing a loved one to suicide. . . no one blames you. . . and you feel no sense of shame because everyone in the room is just like you. It's the first time you feel this way around others, even family members. Because when you are with family members, there is little discussion of the pain. So here you are around strangers, feeling safe, and having lots of discussion—about the pain! So leaving that safety net becomes difficult.

Once everyone finally left, the three of us sat in the lobby and talked about how this needed to be done on an annual basis in other parts of the country. So, we took our show on the road. NOPCAS, the National Organization for People of Color Against Suicide was founded. It is the only minority national organization whose primary focus is suicide prevention in this country. Please visit our website at http://www.nopcas.com.

♥

Chapter

4

Suicide Prevention in the Black Community

Depression And Mental Illness •Black Families
•Religion And Suicide In Black Communities
•Black Organizations •Black-Specific Survivors
Of Suicide Groups (Bssos) •The Collective
Strengths Of Black People

Depression and Mental Illness

The causes of suicide are many and varied.
Suicide is a process, a complicated process that
ends with the act of someone's taking his or her
life. How often have you heard that a person killed
himself, or herself, because of a lost job, wayward
spouse, denial of an expected professional
advancement, or the threat of a sudden severance
of a relationship? These are precipitating events,
but not the causes of suicide. The process of suicide
is far more complicated than one single event.
Depression is the psychiatric diagnosis and the
psychological state most commonly associated with
suicide. Depression affects millions of people. For
a variety of reasons, most black people with
depression and other psychological problems are
going undiagnosed, misdiagnosed and untreated.

The lack of adequate diagnosis and treatment is partly due to family members and friends not recognizing the common signs and symptoms of depression and not seeking professional help in a timely manner. Significant changes in behavior like inability to sleep or sleeping too much; lack of energy; poor appetite, or eating too much, are common symptoms of depression. Feelings of sadness for long periods of time, irritability and restlessness; an inability to think clearly, or to concentrate are also signs of depression. To these I add feelings of sadness, worthlessness or guilt, loss of interest in, and withdrawal from one's usual activities, and repeated thoughts of death or suicide. I also add chronic pain and other physical problems where treatment is ignored, increased risk-taking behavior, including reckless driving, substance abuse, and combativeness as symptoms of depression. We can add many others to these symptoms, including combinations of those listed.

It is extremely important for black people to realize and accept the fact that depression is a mental illness that affects thousands of black people. More importantly, health professionals can treat a mental illness with medication and talk therapy (counseling and psychotherapy). Black people must also come to terms with the fact that suicide is a part of the black culture in America. We can no longer deny the reality of suicide in the black community. The response to those who show signs and symptoms of depression and suicidal behavior must be immediate. One must be concerned, caring, compassionate, and armed with knowledge. Let us prepare to go help save lives.

Black Families

We often view black families as a close-knit group. This group often not only includes the core family, parents and siblings, but also an extended family as well. The extended family may include grandparents, uncles, aunts and cousins. The black family often encompasses more than just blood relatives and relatives by marriage; it sometimes includes neighbors and friends.

Historically, black families have banded together, first for survival and then for support of each other. Prior to the Civil Rights Movement of the 1960s, black people had a clearly defined enemy, "the white power structure," which imposed many limitations on us through laws of segregation and deep-seated customs of discrimination. However, as things became less segregated during the 1960s and 1970s, the more obvious signs of discrimination—"colored" or "Negro" entrance and white-only signs were removed from public facilities—there seemed to have been a false sense of white acceptance of black people. This false sense of acceptance may have contributed to a decline in black cohesiveness.

Black families must restore and enhance the cohesiveness of the past to help insulate us, to some extent, from suicide. A large number of black people have begun this process and are returning "home" to the Southern states where they were born and where they have a sense of their roots. Other ways to enhance a feeling of belonging is through family reunions, annual alumni meetings of former all-black high schools and reunions at historically black colleges and universities. Membership in primarily black social and professional organizations also fosters and continues black cohesiveness. For my purposes, the black church with its various denominations, customs, and traditions is also an agent of cohesiveness.

Religion and Suicide in Black Communities

For years, black people believed that the church had the answer to all of their questions and the solutions to all of their problems. The black church has been the cornerstone of black survival. The church has a unique opportunity to continue in that vein in the prevention of black suicide.

Black people are far more likely to go to a minister, or to another church member with their problems of depression, or suicide concerns than to a mental health professional. In order for the clergy to respond to persons with mental health problems like depression, or suicidal concerns, appropriately, they must become more knowledgeable in these areas. They must become more familiar with mental health professionals and mental health facilities in their respective communities where they can refer depressed or suicidal individuals.

In his 1992 book, *Religion and Suicide in the African-American Community,* Kevin Early interviewed black ministers in a Southern city to get their views and attitudes of the black church toward suicide. "The pastors condemn suicide and define it as so alien to the black experience that even contemplating suicide is excluded as contradictory to what it means to be black. Whites may do it, but blacks do not" (p. 45).

Given the black church's reluctance to acknowledge suicide as a reality, I raise the question of its effectiveness as a buffer to black suicide. How willing would black people be to go to the black church for help with a problem about which the church is in a state of denial? The reality is that there are thousands of black suicides each year, leaving behind an even greater number of survivors. How effective can the black church be in reducing the number of suicides, or in assisting the survivors if the church does not accept the reality of suicide?

The black church must become a major force in suicide prevention in the black community. However, if the church is to become more helpful in the area of suicide prevention, it must provide more black ministers and other faith-based leaders with appropriate education and training about suicidal behaviors. This training would include information regarding suicide gestures, suicide attempts and completed suicides, direct and indirect suicides, substance abuse, neglected health care, and victim-precipitated suicide. In addition, of course, they must become informed of available information on depression—its signs and symptoms, and sources for help.

In order to prevent suicide, it is imperative that black medical professionals, black mental health professionals and black church leaders work together in helping black people see the relationship between religion and medicine, between religion and mental health, between religion and suicide prevention. Fortunately, there has been a relatively new movement in that direction. Sherry Davis Molock, a psychologist and minister, is doing research in this area along with some others. It is from the combined and cooperative efforts of these groups that the largest number of black people can be reached in the education, understanding and the prevention of Black suicide.

Black Organizations

One of the best ways to work toward reducing the number of black suicides is to educate black people about this tragic reality. This education can be done by the many grassroots and well-known national black organizations. Through these organizations, we can educate, inform and spread information throughout the black community. This information would include the signs and symptoms of someone who may be suicidal, the role of depression, its signs and symptoms, as well as where in the community a person could go for help.

We need to ensure that suicide hotlines and crisis center employees are culturally sensitive in responding to black people who are seeking information, or who may be in crisis. A significant number of people who commit suicide visit a medical doctor's office within months of their suicide. Medical associations can address the issues of depression, suicidal behaviors and suicide itself at their meetings to better inform and educate their members in recognizing and treating depressed and suicidal black patients.

A more informal, yet very significant, way of working toward educating the public about the problem of suicide would be through barbershops, beauty shops and pool halls. Persons employed in these establishments could be trained to recognize and appropriately respond when a suicide issue presents itself in their place of business.

Black-Specific Survivors of Suicide Groups (BSSOS)

It is estimated that each suicide intimately affects at least six other people who may be called suicide survivors. Among black people with large extended families, I believe that the number is much higher than six. Based on the numbers of black suicides each year, there are thousands of grieving black survivors left behind. Seeking help from an appropriate professional is the primary recommendation for survivors. For many, another way of working through their grief is by attending Survivors of Suicide groups (SOS).

Studies as well as anecdotal data gathered in the mid-90s indicate that many black survivors are reluctant to attend such groups. Because white professionals generally lead the groups and most of the group members are white, black survivors believe that SOS groups will *not* meet their needs. This reluctance to attend is often generated by the white group leader's misunderstanding of black culture in general, and most importantly, the culture's religious concepts and ways of grieving. This is not to say that black people cannot derive some benefit from such groups. This type of group therapy will probably benefit the survivor. No group participation at all has few benefits.

There is a great need for black-specific survivors of suicide groups (BSSOSG) led by blacks. Fortunately, these groups are available. They reduce the cultural gaps and provide an environment for black group members to express themselves more freely and with a greater degree of confidence that what they say, and how they express their emotions will be understood and accepted.

The Collective Strengths of Black People

One of the most important ways of helping to reduce the number of black suicides is to build upon our ancestry strengths as black people. A good way of doing this is by maintaining and enhancing intergenerational connectedness, which is a multifaceted phenomenon. A bond exists between all black people. However, many black Americans deny the existence of this bond and believe that because of the Civil Rights Movement of the 1960s and 1970s whites now view and accept them for what they have to offer, irrespective of their race. Those who accept this faulty premise are doomed to failure in many areas of their lives. Racism affects the lives of all black people and is a major cause of stress for black people. It continues to affect our mental and physical health on a daily basis. One way of enhancing immunity to suicide is by building on one's individual and ethnic strength.

One way we can garner ethnic strength is through intergenerational connectedness—a spirit, a force, which connects us to our ancestors and the many struggles they endured in order to survive. That strength must be absorbed and used by the present generation to grow and to improve the conditions of all black people. This generation must continue to build upon their ancestors' accomplishments and to pass on their positive black attributes to the children and the younger generations so they can continue black racial pride and progress.

Whether contemporary blacks accept it or not, they are victims of humiliation, degradation, and attempted dehumanization by the institution of slavery. Racism continues to be far more pervasive than many of us would like to believe. In *Lay My Burden Down*, authors Alvin Poussaint and Amy Alexander clearly reveal that slavery and racism continue to affect black lives. And Joy Degruy Leary discusses the impact of slavery and racism on black people in detail in *Post Traumatic Slave Syndrome*.

It appears at times that black people are trying to forget about slavery and its ensuing degradation. We should not forget it, or dismiss it simply as a tragedy best left in the past. While present-day whites benefit from slavery, present-day blacks suffer from the institution of slavery. It has left black people with psychological scars and emotional pain that still affect their lives.

The older generations must continue to teach and enlighten the younger generation about black history and to support and encourage them to pass that history on to those who follow them. In so doing, black people will stop using the white cultural standards as their measurement of success, or completeness as a human being. As black people continue to embrace and incorporate the richness and many accomplishments of their ancestors, they will become wiser, healthier and stronger as an ethnic group. Developing more positive self-concepts and levels of self-esteem will serve as deterrents to suicide and other forms of individual and racial self-destruction.

Where to go for Help

The following resources are available if you, or someone you know, is showing signs of suicidal behaviors:

Local Mental Health Center or Crisis Center (Yellow Pages)

National Suicide Hotline (1-800-784-2433)

National Suicide Prevention Lifeline (1-800-273-8255)

National Suicide Deaf Hotline (1-800-799-4889)

Your Family Physician

Hospital Emergency Room

Police Emergency (911)

Minister, Priest, Rabbi, Imam or other Religious Leaders

Friend or Family Member

Survivors of Suicide Groups

Postscript

Most books have a beginning, middle, and end. This is not that type of book. I want to bring black suicide out of the closet. I want this book, no matter its form, to help black people to start working more openly, and more directly, in educating themselves on the pervasiveness of suicides. Perhaps we can begin to reduce significantly the number of black suicides.

We must view suicide as one spoke in a wheel of destructive behaviors that include drug addiction, alcoholism, abusive use of prescription medication, and black-on-black crimes—assaults, domestic violence and homicides. Other spokes in the wheel of destructive behavior are health-related issues like obesity and high-risk sexual behavior. These behaviors and others may result in prolonged stress, which can be harmful to the individual as well as family members, friends, neighbors and co-workers.

Black suicide is a reality; yes, black people do kill themselves and far more frequently than most of us realize. Depression is the most common psychological state associated with suicide. Mental health professionals can treat depression. It is impossible for us to prevent all black suicides, but we must try. We have to publicize within the black community and its many institutions, organizations and social groups, as well as to both physical and mental health providers that black suicide is real. From a spiritual point, we must acknowledge and strengthen our common bonds of love and respect for each other, especially our elders. We are a resilient people; we had to be in order to survive the transplantation from Africa to the United States and the resulting slavery, oppression, segregation, discrimination and attempted dehumanization after our arrival.

We also share the common bond of a desire to be ourselves, "real people," not shadows of another people. In his book, *In the Beginning Even the Rat Was White,* Robert Guthrie, a black psychologist, says that whites see other ethnic groups as fellow human beings, but human beings who are inferior to them. On the other hand, white people see black people as being a sub-human race. Therein is their justification for having enslaved us in the past and for viewing us as less than equal in the present. These treatments, especially during slavery, have caused severe emotional pain and left profound psychological scars that black people on various levels of consciousness continue to deal with to this day.

In spite of this long history of inhumane treatment, we have survived and we will continue to do so. Our roots, our strengths, our hope, and our resolve guarantee that we will not only survive, we will advance and thrive.

Selected Bibliography

Barnes, Donna Holland. "The Aftermath of Suicide Among African American." *Journal of Black Psychology*, Vol. 32 No. 3 August 2006.

Barksdale, Crystal, Matlin, Samatha, Molock, Sherry Davis and Puri, Rupa. "Relationship Between Religious Coping and Suicidal Behavior Among African American Adolescents." *Journal of Black Psychology*, Vol. 32 No. 3 August 2006.

Breed, Warren. "The Negro and Fatalistic Suicide," *Pacific Sociological Review,* 1970, 13 56-162

Crosby, Alex E., and Molock, Sherry Davis. "Introduction: Suicidal Behavior In The African American Community."*Journal of Psychology* Vol. 32 No. 3 August 2006.

Davis, Robert. "Black Suicide in the Seventies," *Suicide and Life Threatening Behavior*. Fall 1979: Vol. 9 No. 3 131-140l.

Dennis, R., and Kirk, A., "The Use of Crisis Centers by the Black Populations". Suicide and Life Threatening Behavior, Vol. 6 No. 2 101-105. Summer 1976.

Durkheim, Emile. *Suicide*. Translated by John A. Spaulding and George Simpson. New York: The Free Press, 1951.

Early, Kevin E. *Religion and Suicide in the African-American Community*, Connecticut: Greenwood Press,1994.

Freud, Sigmund. "Mourning and Melancholia, (1917)," in *Collective Papers*. Vol. IV. New York: Basic Books, 152-170.

Freud, Sigmund. *The Ego and the Id*, (1923). Translated by Joan Riviere. New York: W.W. Norton and Co., Inc., 1962.

Gibbs, Jack P. & Martin, Walter T. *Status Integration and Suicide: A*

Sociological Study. Oregon: University of Oregon, 1964.

Guthrie, Robert V. *Even the Rat Was White: A Historical View of Psychology*, Boston: Allyn & Bacon,1976.

Hendin, Herbert. *Black Suicide*. New York: Basic Books, Inc., 1969.

Henry, Andrew F. & Short, James F. "Suicide and Homicide: Some Economic," *Sociological And Psychological Aspects of Aggression*. Glencoe, Ill: The Free Press, 1954.

Joe, Sean. "Explaining Changes In The Patterns of Black Suicide in the United States From 1981 to 202: An Age, Cohort, and Period Analysis". *Journal of Black Psychology*, August 2006: Vol. 32 No. 3.

Karon, Bertram P. "Suicidal Tendency as the Wish to Hurt Someone Else, and Resulting Treatment Techniques," *Journal of Individual Psychology*, 1964: 20,206-212.

Kirk, Alton R. "Has the Color of the Rat Really Changed?" Reviewp of Guthrie, Robert V. "Even the Rat Was White: A Historical View of Psychology." *Contemporary Psychology*. July 1978: Vol. 23 No. 7 500-501.

Kirk, Alton R. and Zucker, Robert A. "Some Socio-Psychological Factors in Attempted Suicide Among Urban Black Males," *Suicide and Life Threatening Behavior*. 1979.

Kirk, Alton R. "Black Homicide," Chapter in Danto, Bruce L., Bruchans, John, and Kutsher, Austin W. *The Human Side of Homicide*. New York: Columbia University Press, 1982.

Kirk, Alton R. Review of Early, Kevin E. "Religion and Suicide in the African- American Community," *Suicide and Life Threatening Behavior*. Summer 1994: Vol. 24 No. 2 201-202.

Kirk, Alton R. "Suicide: A Stress Component in Black Males," *Urban Health* September 1977: Vol. 6 No.6.

Leary, Joy Degruy (2005). *Post Traumatic Slave Syndrome: American's Legacy of Enduring Injury and Healing*. Milwaukee: Uptone Press, 2005

Maris, Ronald W. *Social Forces in Urban Suicide*, Homewood, IL: The Free Press, 1969.

Menninger, Karl A. *Man Against Himself*. New York: Harcourt, Brace and Co., 1938.

Prudhomme, C. "The Problem of Suicide in the American Negro," *Psychoanalytic Review*. 1938: 25 187-204,373-391.

Poussaint, Alvin E. & Alexander, Amy. *Lay My Burden Down—Unraveling*

Suicide and Mental Health Crisis Among African-Americans, Boston: Beacon Press, 2000.

Robinson, Edwin Arlington. "Richard Cory" in *Collected Poems of Edwin Arlington Robinson*. New York: The Macmillan Company, 1935 and 1937.

Rucker, Camille M. "How to Prevent Suicide," *Ebony*. December 1976, p 128.

Seiden, Richard H. "We're Driving Young Blacks to Suicide". *Psychology Today*, 1970: 24-28.

Seiden, Richard H. "Why are Suicides of Young Blacks Increasing?", *HSMH Health Report*, No. 87, January, 1972: 3-8.

U.S. Public Health Service. *The Surgeon General's Call To Action To Prevent Suicide*. Washington, Dc: 1999.

Wright, Bobby. *Black Suicide—Lynching By Any Other Name Is Still Lynching*, 1980.